D1637471

Behaviour and Immunity

Behaviour

and

Immunity

Editor

Alan J. Husband

Associate Professor of Immunology
Faculty of Medicine
University of Newcastle
Newcastle, N.S.W., Australia

CRC Press
Boca Raton Ann Arbor London

Library of Congress Cataloging-in-Publication Data

Behaviour and immunity / editor, Alan J. Husband.
    p.   cm.
    Contains papers presented at a scientific meeting of the Australian Behavioural Immunology Group held on Nov. 19, 1990.
    Includes bibliographical references and index.
    ISBN 0-8493-0199-8
    1. Neuroimmunology--Congresses. 2. Psychoneuroimmunology--Congresses. I. Husband, Alan J., 1949-   II. Australian Behavioural Immunology Group.
    [DNLM: 1. Central Nervous System--physiology-- congresses. 2. Conditioning (Psychology)--congresses. 3. Immune System--physiology--congresses. 4. Psychoneuroimmunology--congresses.   WL 103 B4175 1990]
QP56.47.B44   1991
616.07'9--dc20
DNLM/DLC
for Library of Congress   91-35318
                                                   CIP

This book represents information obtained from authentic and highly regarded sources. Reprinted material is quoted with permission, and sources are indicated. A wide variety of references are listed. Every reasonable effort has been made to give reliable data and information, but the authors and the publisher cannot assume responsibility for the validity of all materials or for the consequences of their use.

All rights reserved. This book, or any parts thereof, may not be reproduced in any form without written consent from the publisher.

Direct all inquiries to CRC Press, Inc., 2000 Corporate Blvd., N.W., Boca Raton, Florida, 33431.

© 1992 by CRC Press, Inc.

International Standard Book Number 0-8493-0199-8

Library of Congress Card Number 91-35318

Printed in the United States of America 1 2 3 4 5 6 7 8 9 0

PREFACE

There has been a long standing perception that state of mind and behavioural patterns have an impact on general health. How often do we hear it said that becoming tired and rundown renders us more prone to infection, or the more sinister advice that modern living creates stresses which generate within us an adaptive response which increases susceptibility to illness? We hear anecdotal evidence of remarkable remissions from cancer through positive thinking and imagery. How much of this is folklore and fantasy or is there a link between the psyche and immune sentinel?

The area of Psychoimmunology is a new frontier in biomedical research which probes the way in which the central nervous system and the immune system interact. A large body of data is now accumulating to confirm that, contrary to the traditional view of the immune system as a self-regulating network of cells and molecules, the activities of the central nervous system have profound influence on immune function. There is now intense interest in the parameters which govern these interactions, the mediators involved and the extent to which health and well being are modified by behaviour. The impact of these studies on veterinary and human health management will be profound. Avoidance of stress and adequate sleep are now being placed high on the health agenda. There is now a perceived role for deliberate manipulations of behavioural responses, for instance through learned associations (conditioning), to modify immune function. By these techniques the effects of a useful drug could be enhanced, or the required dosage of a toxic drug reduced, by harnessing the potential of the brain to manipulate the immune system to re-enlist the effects of those drugs when given in association with a sensory cue. Personality profiles are now being linked to defined disease patterns. Thus the physician of the future may add to his list of pills and potions, a set of behavioural recommendations for the treatment of illness.

The Australian Behavioural Immunology Group was established in response to the need to provide a forum for presentation of data and exchange of ideas regarding the concept of brain, behaviour and immunity. The papers presented at the first scientific meeting of the Group are presented in this volume representing the state of the art in a number of areas where these interactions have been studied. This meeting was made possible by the generous support of a number of organizations:

Sandoz Australia Pty Ltd
The Hunter Medical Research Co-operative Ltd, Newcastle, Australia
The Faculty of Medicine of the University of Newcastle, Australia

I am also grateful to the organizing committee, Dr Roger Bartrop, Professor Claude Bernard, Dr Richard Brown, Ms Diane Bull, Dr Maryann Gauci, Professor Maurice King, Dr Peter Pfister, Dr Maryanne O'Donnell, and Dr Manfred Schedlowski, who contributed to the success of this meeting. We look forward to continued progress in this important area of scientific endeavour.

Alan J. Husband, Ph.D, FASM.

ABSTRACT

This volume contains papers presented at a scientific meeting of the The Australian Behavioural Immunology Group (November 10, 1990, Newcastle, NSW, Australia), representing current research in the area of behavioural and central nervous system effects on immune function. This is a new frontier in biomedical research. A large body of data is now accumulating to confirm that, contrary to the traditional view of the immune system as a self-regulating network of cells and molecules, the activities of the central nervous system have profound influence on immune function. There is now intense interest in the parameters which govern these interactions, the mediators involved, and the extent to which health and well-being are modified by behaviour. The impact of these studies on veterinary and human health management will be profound. Avoidance of stress and adequate sleep are now being placed high on the health agenda. There is now a perceived role for deliberate manipulations of behavioural responses, for instance through learned associations (conditioning), to modify immune function. By these techniques the effects of a useful drug could be enhanced, or the required dosage of a toxic drug reduced, by harnessing the potential of the brain to manipulate the immune system to re-enlist the effects of those drugs when given in association whith a sensory cue. Personality profiles are now being linked to defined disease patterns. The clinical implications of this research are that the physician of the future may add to his list of pills and potions, a set of behavioural recommendations for the treatment of illness.

THE EDITOR

Alan J. Husband is Associate Professor in Immunology in the Faculty of Medicine at the University of Newcastle in Australia. Dr. Husband graduated from the University of Sydney with an honours degree in Agricultural Science in 1972 and was awarded a PhD degree from the same university in 1975 for studies of immunity in ruminants. After post-doctoral studies at the Sir William Dunn School of Pathology at the University of Oxford, he returned to Australia in 1977 to the position of Research Scientist and head of the Immunology section of the New South Wales State Department of Agriculture Central Veterinary Laboratories. In 1980 he accepted his current appointment at the University of Newcastle.

Dr. Husband is a Fellow of the Australian Society for Microbiology and member of the Australian Society for Immunology, the Australian Society for Medical Research and the American Association of Immunologists. He has authored in excess of 100 scientific publications, mostly in the area of mucosal immune defence, but since 1982 has developed additional interests in the emerging area of psychoimmunology, the roles of behaviour and the central nervous system in immunity. He was one of the foundation members of the Australian Behavioural Immunology Group and is currently the National Convenor of that organisation.

TABLE OF CONTENTS

IV. Life Events, Exercise and Immunity

V. Impact of Psychoimmunology in Clinical Medicine

I. Biochemistry, Neurophysiology and

Endocrinology of CNS-Immune Interactions

BRAIN IMMUNE PATHWAYS REGULATING IMMUNOLOGICAL FUNCTION AND CONDITIONED IMMUNE RESPONSES

Arnold H. Greenberg, Richard Brown, Zuo Li and Dennis G. Dyck

Manitoba Institute of Cell Biology and the Department of Psychology
University of Manitoba, 100 Olivia Street, Winnipeg, MB, Canada R3E OV9

I. ABSTRACT

A basic assumption of the study of CNS-immune interactions is that the immune system can signal the brain and that the brain can subsequently modify peripheral immune function. We hypothesized that Pavlovian conditioning of immunity is mediated by these immunomodulatory CNS signals. The best described pathway from the immune system to the CNS is mediated by the lymphokine interleukin-l (IL-1). IL-1 can stimulate the release of ACTH from pituitary and increase body temperature through its effects on central thermoregulatory centers. We have examined the conditionability of this pathway and have shown that IL-1 induced activation of the pituitary-adrenal axis and pyrexic responses can be conditioned by classical Pavlovian conditioning procedures using taste and olfactory cues.

Based on this model, it was predicted that IL-1 would not only stimulate the brain, but would also modify peripheral immune function through its direct action on the brain. Intracerebroventricular (ICV) injection of IL-1 at doses which were steriodogenic resulted in the suppression of the splenic macrophage IL-1 secretion following in vitro stimulation. Both adrenalectomy (ADX) and surgical sympathectomy (SX) of the spleen prevented the macrophage suppressive signals of ICV IL-1. The combination of ADX and SX produced potent macrophage stimulatory effects, arguing that both the hypothalamic-pituitary-adrenal axis and the sympathetic nervous system can regulate peripheral immune function from the brain.

The existence of a regulatory pathway from the immune system to the CNS and back to the immune system suggests that the phenomena of conditioning of immune responses may be explained through the action of classical immunoregulatory lymphokines such as IL-1 on humoral and neural regulatory pathways.

II. INTRODUCTION

Bi-directional communication between the central nervous system and the immune system was first proposed by Besedovsky and colleagues.[1-3] In their model, products of the immune system released from stimulated immune cells signal the brain which consequently induced a response that down-regulated immune function. Most prominent of the lymphokines to produce central effects is interleukin-l.[4] IL-1 is a 17.5 kd peptide of two forms, named IL-

1α and IL-1β, originating primarily from activated macrophages which has a primary role in amplification of T cell responses and in acute phase reactions during infections. IL-1 has been shown to induce fever and slow wave sleep, alter hypothalamic norepinephrine turnover and release hypothalamic corticotropin releasing factor (CRF) and ACTH.[3,5-8] Many of these responses are similar to those seen during immune responses.[9,10] Recent evidence indicates that IL-1 can affect the metabolism of norepinephrine (NE) as reflected by the increasing ratio of MHPG to NE.[8] The hypothalamus and in particular the paraventricular hypothalamic nucleus (PVN) appears to play an important role in CRF release and is a target for IL-1 and antigen induced alteration in NE metabolism and increased electrical activity.[8,11,12] An immune response to sheep erythrocytes (SRBC) and intraperitoneal injection of IL-1 also affects the level of NE, serotonin and serotonin metabolites in other brain areas.[12] In addition, forebrain areas providing direct and indirect input to the hypothalamus, such as the septal and hippocampal areas, have been implicated in the control of immune function,[13] are major target areas for corticosterone[14] and contain IL-1 receptors.[15] Finally, the lateral septal area has been shown to be the site of action for the anti-pyretic effects of α-MSH in rabbits made febrile by the IL-1 injection (Lipton, 1988). While it is not clear that IL-1 can cross the blood brain barrier, there are areas close to the hypothalamus which are free of this constraint. A small amount of IL-1 or a fragment may cross these areas and autoinduce further production of IL-1 or an intermediate which can act as a transmitter to hypothalamic nuclei. It has been demonstrated that IL-1 immunoreactive fibers innervate the hypothalamus, that it is present in cell bodies in the hypothalamus and that IL-1 receptors are also located in the hypothalamus.[15,16].

The impact of CNS signalling on various components of the immune system has been demonstrated through various behavioral conditioning studies.[17-23] The procedure in these studies involves pairing a distinctive environmental stimulus (conditional stimulus; CS) with a potent immunomodulatory agent (unconditional stimulus; UCS). Conditioning is typically inferred on the basis of an altered immune response to a later presentation of the CS (conditioned response; CR) although a modified systemic response (UR) to a cued presentation of a drug after repeated cue-drug pairings (e.g. conditioned tolerance) has also been interpreted as evidence for conditioning.[20,21] In the latter instance, the inference of an associative process is warranted only if the altered UCR is context-specific to cues paired with the UCS, and additionally demonstrates a sensitivity to known conditioning procedures such as extinction or CS pre-exposure.

The most popular conditioning procedure that has been applied to the modification of immune function is the taste aversion model. The pairing of taste with different illness-inducing agents results in an avoidance of the solution containing the novel taste (e.g. saccharin). Pairing with LiCl also produces conditioned taste aversion.[24] Most experiments on taste aversion learning have used an immunosuppressive drug, cyclophosphamide, and shown that the re-exposure to the taste cue re-elicits the immunosuppressive response. Using this model, conditioned immunosuppression has been observed for antibody responses[17] and CTL induction.[25] The taste aversion model has recently been used to condition the release of mast cell specific proteases.[19] These conditioned responses appear to have biological significance and can alter the outcome of autoimmune disease in NZB mice,[17] GVH disease,[26] and tumor immunity.[18]

Immunopharmacological conditioning work from our laboratory on the tolerance of poly I:C induced NK cell activation[20] has also been immunosuppressive in nature. Poly I:C stimulates macrophage IL-1 secretion, and IL-1 has a thermoregulatory pyrexic effect and can stimulate ACTH and corticosterone secretion. We subsequently examined the conditionability of poly I:C induced pyrexic responses. In these studies we have shown that in mice, poly I:C induced pyrexic responses are conditionable to odor cues and the CR is a hypothermic response.[27]

Another prediction of the tolerance model is that poly I:C induced ACTH and glucocorticoid responses should be immunosuppressive. This was subsequently examined by directly stimulating ACTH release through intracerebroventricular administration of recombinant IL-1β, a procedure that avoids the complicating features of peripheral IL-1 effects on immune function.

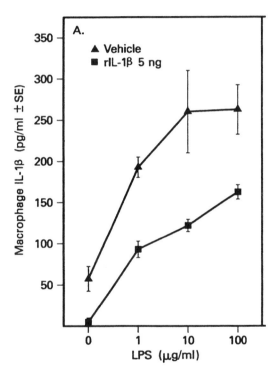

Figure 1: Suppression of splenic macrophage IL-1 production by ICV injection of 5 ng recombinant IL-1β (F) (1.32) = 9.56, p < 0.01). Spleens were collected 2 hrs post-injection. N = 5 rats/group. Macrophages recovered from spleens were stimulated in vitro with LPS at the dose indicated. From Brown et al.[30]

III. INTRACEREBROVENTRICULAR IL-1 INDUCES IMMUNOSUPPRESSION VIA ADRENAL AND SYMPATHETIC AUTONOMIC PATHWAYS.

The hypothesis that the central effects of IL-1 influence peripheral immune function has been tested by Sundar et al.[28] and Weiss et al.[29] and our laboratory.[30] These experiments use the infusion of IL-1β into the lateral ventricle, subsequently monitoring modifications in peripheral immunity. The work of Sundar et al.[28] identified an immunosuppressive effect on NK cell activity, PHA responsiveness and IL-2 production following PHA stimulation in animals given ICV IL-1 between the doses of 50 and 200 pg. This effect could be blocked by α-MSH but was only partially reversed by adrenalectomy.

In experiments from our laboratory, at doses between 5 and 100 ng of rIL-1β infused ICV, a suppression of splenic macrophage secretion of IL-1 in response to LPS stimulation was observed (Fig. 1) and was coincidental with increases in the secretion of ACTH and corticosterone. Adrenalectomy completely reversed the suppressive effect of central IL-1 and cutting the splenic nerve was as effective as adrenalectomy. Combined nerve section and adrenalectomy resulted in an enhanced responsiveness of LPS stimulated macrophages (Fig. 2). Sundar et al.[28] found that injection of IL-1 into the cisterna magna or intraperitoneally was ineffective, and we have demonstrated that the equivalent dose of IL-1 injected intraperitoneally stimulated rather than suppressed macrophage function. Taken together, these data argue that ICV injections of IL-1 activates two immunosuppressive pathways, pituitary ACTH which releases circulating glucocorticoids, as well as a neural sympathetic signal which can effect splenic lymphocyte and macrophage function. The latter is consistent with the studies of Felten et al.[31] who have demonstrated the sympathetic innervation of the spleen and nerve contact with both T cells and macrophages.

IV. CONDITIONING OF IL-1 RESPONSES

Corticosterone is a well known immunosuppressant and anti-inflammatory steroid hormone that is produced in response to immune stimulation[32,33] and is capable of blocking macrophage secretion of IL-1.[34] This has led to the proposal that this CNS-immune pathway operates as a negative feedback mechanism to immune activation.[3,35] Since all but a few examples of conditioned immunopharmacologic effects are immunosuppressive,[17,18,20,21,25,36] and corticosterone production can be conditioned,[37] it is possible that IL-1 induced corticosterone responses are subject to modification by Pavlovian conditioning procedures. We have examined whether recombinant IL-1β-induced corticosterone production could be conditioned to cues paired with intraperitoneal administration of the peptide. We utilized a Pavlovian conditioning procedure that has been used successfully to modify immune responses by many other groups based on the work of Ader and Cohen who established that exposure of rats to saccharin and the immunosuppressive drug, cyclophosphamide leads to the elicitation of a cyclophosphamide-like immunosuppressive response following re-exposure of animals to saccharin in their drinking water. In addition, we have recently used an odor conditioning protocol to condition NK cell responses. Odor is a potent cue for conditioned tolerance or suppression of poly I:C-induced NK cell responses.[20,21]

We have found evidence for conditioning of rIL-1β-induced corticosterone secretion using the taste aversion conditioning model (Fig. 3) as well as odor conditioning using three

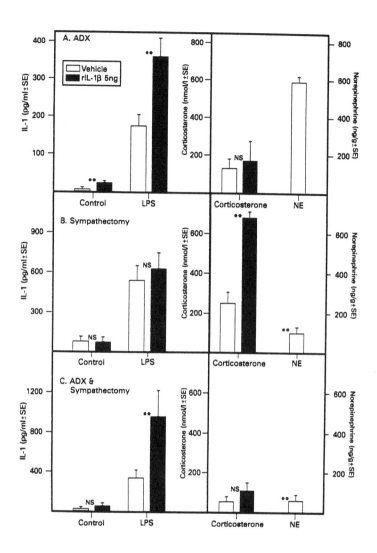

Figure 2: Effect of 5 ng recombinant IL-1β or saline ICV on splenic macrophage IL-1 production with or without LPS stimulation. (A) ADX (adrenolectomy), (B) splenic nerve section and (C) ADX plus splenic nerve section. Macrophages were cultured with 10 mg of LPS as in Figure 1. Rats receive 5 ng IL-1β ICV ( ). or saline ( ) ICV. Spleens were assayed for norepinephrine content and serum assayed for corticosterone on each animal to confirm the success of the adrenylectomy in nerve section. ** = p < 0.01, * = p < 0.05. NS, not significant; NE, norepinephrine; N = 5-8 rats/group. From Brown et al.[30]

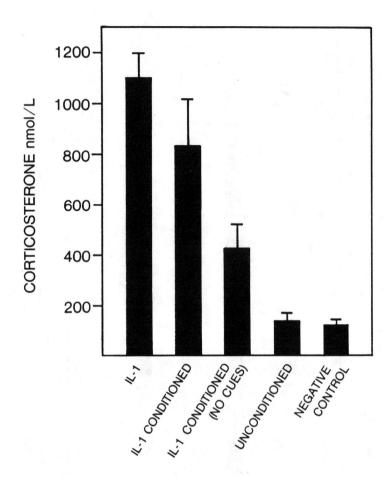

Figure 3: Taste aversion conditioning protocol measuring serum corticosterone levels 2 hrs following the re-exposure to saccharine/lithium chloride conditioning stimulus. IL-1 conditioned mice have significantly higher corticosterone levels than the IL-1 conditioned (no cues), unconditioned and negative control groups. From Dyck et al.[22]

types of cue presentations (saccharin, saccharin and LiCl, odor).[23]

V. A MODEL FOR CNS-IMMUNE INTERACTION IN CONDITIONING

Conditioning is a CNS phenomenon which involves the integration and learning of perceptual and interoceptive signals (CSs) with other physiologically salient events (UCSs). A conditioned immune response requires that following integration of the correct perceptual signal (CS), the CNS associates this with some physiological effects of the immune effects. Thus a response occurs to the CS alone. The mechanisms by which this occurs are not well established, but likely involve both humoral and neural processes mediated via the endocrine system and sympathetic autonomic system which innervates all lymphoid organs.[38-41] The

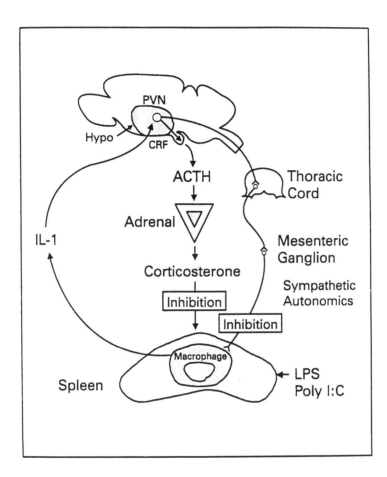

Figure 4: A model for the immune-CNS interaction mediated by IL-1. Evidence for conditioning of this pathway includes the ability to condition both IL-1-induced corticosterone secretion as well as IL-1-induced pyrexic responses. IL-1 mediated regulatory pathways for macrophage stimulation occur through both the ACTH/adrenocorticoid pathway as well as autonomic sympathetics innervating spleen.

possibility that IL-1 can both mediate peripheral immunomodulation via the brain and that this response is conditionable has now been partially tested. IL-1 induced corticosterone responses could thus account for some conditioned immunosuppression phenomena. However, the identification of a functional immunosuppressive pathway via the autonomic sympathetics that can be IL-1 stimulated offers another possible mechanism (Fig. 4). This proposal excludes neither other lymphokines that have CNS effects (e.g. TNF-α, IFN-α, IL-6) nor other pathways by which the cytokines can mediate their peripheral effects. Developing of our understanding of CNS-immune interaction is the key to the further study of the biological basis for conditioning of immune responses, as conditioning must have its biological effects by initiating the recapitulation of these physiological CNS-immune pathways.

VI. ACKNOWLEDGEMENTS

This work was supported by grants from the USPHS 2ROlMH43778-04 and the R.J. Reynolds Co.

VII. REFERENCES

1.   Besedovsky, H.O., del Rey, A.E., Sorkin, E., Da Prada, M., Burri, R. and Honegger, C., The immune response evokes changes in brain non-adrenergic neurons, *Science*, 221, 564, 1983.

2.   Besedovsky, H.O., del Rey, A.E. and Sorkin, E., *Neuroimmunology*, Raven Press, New York, 1984, 445.

3.   Besedovsky, H.O., del Rey, A.E., Sorkin, E. and Dinarello, C.A., Immunoregulatory feedback between interleukin-1 and glucocorticoid hormones, *Science*, 233, 652, 1986.

4.   Dinarello, C.A., Biology of interleukin-1, *FASEB J.*, 2, 108, 1988.

5.   Sapolsky, R., Rivier, C., Yamamoto, G., Plotsky, P. and Vale, W., Interleukin-1 stimulates the secretion of hypothalamic corticotropinreleasing factor, *Science*, 238, 522, 1987.

6.   Tobler, I., Borbely, A.A., Schwyzer, M. and Fontana, A., , *Eur.J.Pharmacol.*, 104, 191, 1984.

7.   Berkenbosch, F., van Oelers, J., del Rey, A.E., Tilders, F. and Besedovsky, H., Corticotropin-releasing factor producing neurons in the rat activated by interleukin-1, *Science*, 238, 524, 1987.

8.   Kabiersch, A., del Rey, A.E., Honegger, C.G. and Besedovsky, H.O., Interleukin-1 induces changes in the rat brain, *Brain Behav.Immun.*, 2, 267, 1988.

9.   Besedovsky, H.0., Sorkin, E., Felix, D. and Haas, H., Hypothalamic changes during the immune response, *Eur.J.Immunol.*, 7, 323, 1977.

10. Besedovsky, H.O., del Rey, A.E., Da Prada, M. and Keller, H.H., Immunoregulation mediated by the sympathetic nervous system, *Cell.Immunol.*, 48, 346, 1979.

11. Saphier, D., Abramsby, O., Mor, G. and Ovadia, H., , *Brain Behav.Immun.*, 1, 40, 1987.

12. Carlson, S.L., Felten, D.L., Livnat, S. and Felten, S.Y., Alterations of monoamines in specific central autonomic nuclei following immunization in mice, *Brain Behav.Immun.*, 1, 52, 1987.

13. Nance, D.M., Hopkins, D.A. and Bieger, D., Re-investigation of the innervation of the thymus gland in mice and rats, *Brain Behav.Immun.*, 1, 134, 1987.

14. McEwen, B.S., Weiss, J.M. and Schwartz, L.S., , *Brain Res.*, 16, 227, 1969.

15. Farrar, W.L., Kilian, P.L., Ruff, M.R., Hill, J.M. and Pert, C.B., Visualization and

characterization of interleukin-1 receptors in brain, *J.Immunol.*, 139, 459, 1987.

16. Breder, C.D., Dinarello, C.A. and Saper, C.B., IL-1 immunoreactive innervation of the human hypothalamus, *Science*, 240, 321, 1988.

17. Ader, R. and Cohen, N., Behaviorally conditioned immunosuppression, *Psychosom.Med.*, 37, 333, 1975.

18. Gorczynski, R.M., Kennedy, M. and Ciampi, A., Cimetidine reverses tumor growth enhancement of plasmocytoma tumors in mice demonstrating conditioned immunosuppression, *J.Immunol.*, 134, 4261, 1985.

19. MacQueen, G., Marshall, J., Perdue, M., Siegel, S. and Bienenstock, J., Pavlovian conditioning of rat mucosal cells to secrete rat mast cell protease II, *Science*, 243, 83, 1989.

20. Dyck, D.G., Greenberg, A.H. and Osachuk, T.A.G., Tolerance to drug-induced (poly I:C) natural killer cell activation: Congruence with a Pavlovian conditioning model, *J.Exp.Psy.:Anim.Beh.Proc.*, 12, 25, 1986.

21. Dyck, D.G., Driedger, S.M., Nemeth, R., Osachuk, T.A.G. and Greenberg, A.H., Conditioned tolerance to drug-induced (poly I:C) natural killer cell activation: Effects of drug-dosage and contextspecificity parameters, *Brain Behav.Immun.*, 1, 251, 1987.

22. Dyck, D.G., Janz, L., Osachuk, T.A.G., Falk, J., Labinsky, J. and Greenberg, A.H., The Pavlovian conditioning of IL-1 induced glucocorticoid secretion, *Brain Behav.Immun.*, 4, 93, 1990.

23. Dyck, D.G. and Greenberg, A.H., Immunopharmacological tolerance as a conditioned response: dissecting the brain-immune pathways, in *Psychoneuroimmunology II*, R.Ader, , N.Cohen, and D.Felton, , Eds., Academic Press, New York, 1990, In press.

24. Garcia, J. and Koelling, R.A., Relation of cue to consequence in avoidance learning, *Psychom.Sci.*, 4, 123, 1966.

25. Gorczynski, R.M., McRae, S. and Kennedy, M., Conditioned immune response associated with allogeneic skin grafts in mice, *J.Immunol.*, 129, 704, 1982.

26. Bovbjerg, D., Ader, R. and Cohen, N., Behaviourally conditioned suppression of a graft-versus-host response, *Proc.Natl.Acad.Sci.USA*, 79, 583, 1982.

27. Dyck, D.G., Osachuk, T.A.G. and Greenberg, A.H., Drug-induced (poly I:C) pyrexic responses: Congruence with a compensatory conditioning analysis, *Psychobiology*, 17, 171, 1989.

28. Sundar, S.K., Becker, K.J., Cierpial, M.A., Carpenter, M.D., Rankin, L.A., Fleener, S.L., Ritchie, J.C., Simson, P.E. and Weiss, J.M., Intracerebroventricular infusion of interleukin 1 rapidly decreases peripheral cellular immune responses, *Proc.Natl.Acad.Sci.USA*, 86, 6398, 1989.

29. Weiss, J.M., Sundar, S.K., Becker, K.J. and Cierpial, M.A., Behavioral and neural influences on cellular immune response: effects of stress and interleukin-1, *J.Clin.Psych.*, 50(Suppl.), 43, 1989.

30. Brown, R., Zuo, L., Vriend, C., Nirula, R., Janz, L., Falk, J., Nance, D., Dyck, D. and Greenberg, A.H., Suppression of splenic macrophage IL-1 secretion following intracerebroventricular injection of interleukin-1β: Evidence for pituitary-adrenal and sympathetic control, *Cell.Immunol.*, 1990.(In Press)

31. Felten, D.L., Ackerman, K.D., Wiegand, S.J. and Felten, S.Y., Noradrenergic sympathetic innervation of the spleen. I. Nerve fibers associated with lymphocytes and macrophages in specific compartments of the splenic white pulp, *J.Neurosci.Res.*, 18, 28, 1987.

32. Besedovsky, H.O., del Rey, A.E., Sorkin, E., Lotz, W. and Schwulera, V., Lymphoid cells produce an immunoregulatory glucocorticoid increasing factor (GIF) acting through the pituitary gland, *Clin.Exp.Immunol.*, 69, 622, 1985.

33. Besedovsky, H.O., del Rey, A.E. and Sorkin, E., Lymphokine containing supernatants from Con-A-stimulated cells increase corticosterone levels, *J.Immunol.*, 126, 385, 1981.

34. Snyder, D.S. and Unanue, E.R., Corticosteroids inhibit murine macrophage Ia expression and interleukin-1 production, *J.Immunol.*, 129, 1803, 1982.

35. del Rey, A.E., Besedovsky, H., Sorkin, E. and Dinarello, C.A., Interleukin-1 and glucocorticoid hormones integrate an immunoregulatory feedback circuit, *Ann.N.Y.Acad.Sci.*, 496, 85, 1987.

36. Kusnecov, A.W., Sivyer, M., King, M.G., Husband, A.J., Cripps, A.W. and Clancy, R.L., Behaviorally conditioned suppression of the immune response by antilymphocyte serum, *J.Immunol.*, 130, 2117, 1983.

37. Ader, R., Conditioned adrenocortical steroid elevation in the rat, *J.Comp.Phys.Psych.*, 90, 1156, 1976.

38. Felten, D., Felten, S.Y., Carlson, S.L., Olschowka, J.A. and Livnat, S., Noradrenergic and peptidergic innervation of lymphoid tissue, *J.Immunol.*, 135, 755, 1985.

39. Felten, D.L., Livnat, S.Y., Carlson, S.L., Bellinger, D.L. and Yeh, P., Sympathetic innervation of lymph nodes in mice, *Brain Res.Bull.*, 13, 693, 1984.

40. Nance, D.M. and Burns, J., Innervation of the spleen in the rat: Evidence for absence of afferent innervation, *Brain Behav.Immun.*, 3, 281, 1989.

41. Williams, J.M., Peterson, R.G., Shea, P.A., Schmedtje, J.F., Bauer, D.C. and Felten, D.L., Sympathetic innervation of murine thymus and spleen: Evidence for a functional link between the nervous and immune systems, *Brain Res.Bull.*, 6, 83, 1981.

IMPLICATIONS OF PSYCHOIMMUNOLOGY FOR MODELS OF THE IMMUNE SYSTEM

Roger J. Booth and Kevin R. Ashbridge

Department of Molecular Medicine, Auckland University School of Medicine, Private Bag, Auckland, New Zealand.

"Other Kings said I was daft to build a castle on the swamp but I did it just the same... just to show 'em. It sank into the swamp. So, I built another one... that sank into the swamp. I built another one... that burned down, fell over and then sank into the swamp... so I built another... and that stayed up!"

- Monty Python and the Holy Grail.

I. ABSTRACT

Neuroimmunology is revealing extensive interconnections between the immune and neuroendocrine systems in terms of common receptors, shared informational molecules such as cytokines and neuropeptides, as well as autonomic nervous effects on immune function. As a result, the boundaries between the immune system and the nervous system are becoming progressively less distinct. Extending these findings, research with a more psycho-immunological emphasis is uncovering associations between immunological parameters and psychological variables such as behavioural and affective states. Self/non-self discrimination at the molecular level has traditionally been considered a fundamental property of the immune system. In view of the extensive and pervasive nature of the psychoneuroimmune network, we propose that immune processes should be reconsidered in a psychoimmune context. We suggest that psychological, neuroendocrine and immunological processes are so intimately linked that they cannot be understood effectively in isolation but together constitute an irreducible dynamic process of self-determination. The self as defined immunologically and the psychological self are therefore mutually generative domains rather than independent constructs. This hypothesis has important implications for the interpretation of immunological phenomena and for the understanding of disease processes.

II. INTRODUCTION

The traditional view of the role of the immune system as a defensive and protective mechanism arose from observations of specific immunity following infection and recovery, and the capacity to stimulate this memory response 'artificially' by vaccination. The central tenet of a 'defence system' model is that of somatic self/non-self discrimmation leading to a system which produces effective responses to foreignness but tolerance (non-responsiveness) to self antigens. Definitions of concepts such as forbidden clones, immunological censorship, and positive or negative selective pressures on repertoire development reflect the defensive orientation of the model. Seminal work in the 1960's and 70's considering anti-idiotypic responses and the appreciation of the pivotal position of MHC determinants in antigen presentation[1-4] extended the model to view the immune system as a recursively self-organising, dynamic cellular and molecular network which identifies foreignness in the context of self.

With the advent of research identifying the extensive interpenetration of immune, endocrine and nervous systems by shared informational molecules (neuropeptides, cytokines and hormones) as well as receptors and other cell surface structures[5-10] came the realisation that the conceptual divisional boundaries around the immune, neuroendocrine systems are largely historical artifacts (Figure 1). Further, a growing body of literature is documenting significant associations between

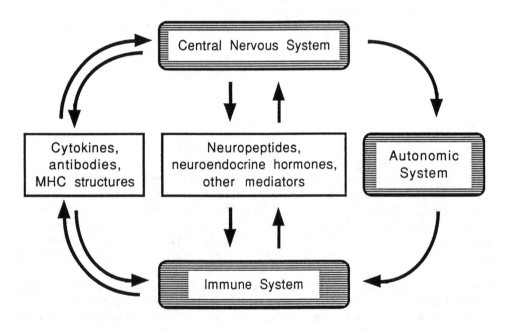

Figure 1. Schematic summary of immune and nervous system interactions.

immunological parameters and psychological variables such as behavioural patterns and affective states.[8-12] Much evidence now exists for viewing the interaction of psychological, neuroendocrine, and immune systems as a complex and integrated whole. Consequently, in order to appreciate the structure and function of the immune system within the whole person, it is necessary to adopt a more expanded view of its boundaries and its interactions. The science of psychoneuroimmunology (PNI) is developing out of the need to address this interaction and integration. However, the complexity, sublety and extent of these often leads to difficulties when using current methods of scientific study and interpretation. This arises partly because the interplay of these systems results in the appearance of irreducible phenomena can not be described simply from the sum of its parts, and the questionable validity of ascribing linear cause-effect pathways among interactive elements of a complex system. Because of the need to maintain system interaction in the study of PNI, a scientific method based solely on reductionism (explanation through successive dissection) and the investigation of mechanism (cause leading to effect) is proving to be inadequate. It is rapidly becoming more useful to consider new approaches and to cultivate new models that still retain the essential elements of successful models used in the study of each system in isolation, but additionally incorporate a better context and perspective from which to understand their interplay. Such understanding centres on a knowledge of what the system as a whole is trying to achieve.

Of considerable importance for the development of ideas in the area of PNI was the recognition of the striking degree of similarity between the immune and nervous systems.[1,3,13] Both systems are involved in the receipt and processing of information - sensory information in the case of the nervous system, while for the immune system it is molecular topological information. Both respond to a diverse range of stimuli and in each case the response is specific for the stimulus. There are a range of available responses and each system adapts its resources to provide those which are appropriate. Neither the immune system nor the nervous system can know in advance what stimuli each is likely to receive during the lifetime of an animal and so the capacity to respond to unexpected stimuli is a fundamental property. Both systems may also remember specific stimuli and modify and tailor subsequent responsiveness. Both the immune and nervous systems are regulated by complex internal networks. These shared qualities led to the suggestion that immunological and neurological responses were metaphorically (and perhaps symbolically) of the same nature.[13]

As shown in Table 1, a number of authors have suggested ways in which the interplay between the immune, neuroendocrine and psychological systems may be perceived. These represent important contributions towards the evolution of new models that address both the physical (molecular) and systemic relationships among mind, brain and immune system. They highlight the informational basis of psychoneuroimmune interactions but, with the exception of Engel's assertion,[14] they explain the nature of the whole system to varying degrees in terms of subsystems or specific contributory components. In effect, they endeavour to understand the behaviour of the whole from the properties of its parts. We believe that any model aspiring to provide a truly novel framework for the PNI network as a whole system must adopt wholeness and indivisibility as fundamental qualities. In order to do this we consider that it is necessary to extend the perceptual framework of the immune system.

III. HYPOTHESIS: SOMATOPSYCHIC[1] DETERMINATION OF SELF

Instead of viewing the immune system as a somatic self/non-self discriminatory mechanism born out of the requirement for protection against foreign invasion, we hypothesise that a central principle from which immune structure and function is derived, is primarily one of somatopsychic determination of self. The immune, neuroendocrine and

---

[1] We have chosen the word *somatopsychic* to avoid the pejorative connotations of *psychosomatic*.

psychological systems together comprise an irreducible self-determining process such that

Table 1. Models of psychoneuroimmune interplay.

MODEL	REFERENCE
The immune system as a sensory organ	Blalock[15]
The immune system as a mobile brain	Blalock and Smith[16]
The neuroendocrine-immune network of informational molecules as the substrate of emotions	Pert, Ruff, Weber and Herkenham[5]
Immune response patterns as vital contributors to the 'biological ergo'	Burgio and Martini[17]
Immune responses as a form of behaviour	Engel[14]

immune responses are not simply reactions to antigenicor psychological stimuli but are integral components of the transformative processes that constitute the somatopsychic life of an individual (Figure 2). In effect, this means that psychological and immunological processes are so intimately linked at all levels that they cannot be understood effectively in isolation, and that the self as defined immunologically and the psychological self are not independent constructs.

IV. MULTI-DIMENSIONALITY OF THE IMMUNE SYSTEM

In terms of molecules, cells and organs, the immune system can be considered as a stable, dynamic, recursive structure which determines the profile of antigenic foreignness with reference to the self antigenic milieu. Our hypothesis implies that this self-referential nature of the immune system is inherently multi-dimensional. It is determined and affected not only by the self-antigenic microcosm but additionally by aspects of the self profiles of other systems which, in turn, it also influences. Thus, the constant appraisal and re-appraisal of antigenic structures encountered by cells and molecules of the immune system constitute vital transformative processes which simultaneously shape both the 'classical' immune response repertoire and the somatopsychic self.

An important implication of this multi-dimensionality is that parallels should be evident among psychological, neuroendocrine and immune system phenomena throughout the life of an individual because each contributes at all stages to the development of the others and self-determination arises as much out of the interaction among these systems as within each system. In support of this, it has been known for some time that an intimate reciprocal

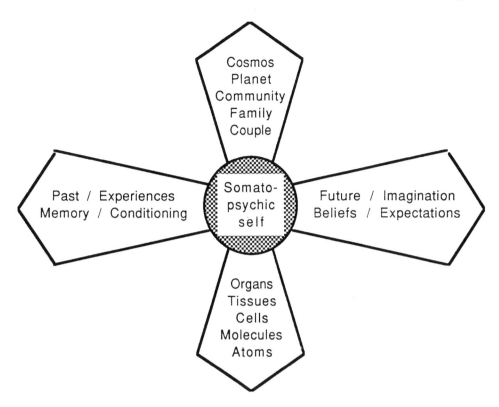

Figure 2. Influences on the somatopsychic-determined self.

relationship exists between the neuroendocrine and immune systems during ontogeny. For example, defective endocrine development (such as occurs in congenitally hypopituitary dwarf mice) is accompanied by impaired B cell and T cell development[18] while conversely, neonatal thymectomy or bursectomy results in neuroendocrine as well as immunological deficiencies.[19] A further example concerns the role of MHC determinants. These have long been recognised as fundamental antigen-presentation structures which govern the nature of epitopes recognised by the immune system. However, recent work[20,21] has revealed that by carrying aromatic chemicals into the urine of rats, soluble MHC molecules define a set of olefactory signals through which individual animals can be identified. Given that olefactory senses are intimately associated with the limbic regions of the brain and that smell and taste senses are potently evocative of strong emotional and other psychological responses,[22] these findings are very much in keeping with the concept of a vital role for MHC in defining the extent or boundaries of the unique psychoimmune self of an individual. The fact that these same structures simultaneously provide elements necessary for antigen recognition highlights the inherent multi-dimensional elegance of immune system structure and function within a somatopsychic self-determination framework.

V. IMMUNE SYSTEM DEVELOPMENT IN A SOMATOPSYCHIC CONTEXT

As the somatopsychic self-determination hypothesis proposes that the nature and behaviour of the immune system will both determine and be determined by psychological and somatic states, parallels should be evident between immunological and psychological events throughout the life of an individual. As a general observation, childhood and adolescence are times when there is growth and development of diverse patterns of response both psychologically and immunologically which contribute to the definition of a unique self. The adult years are when the potentials of the established response patterns are explored and refined, while old age is characterised as a period of involution and preparation for death. Considering the neonatal period more specifically from immunological and psychological perspectives reveals some potentially instructive similarities. The immune systems of neonates are generally regarded as being immature relative to those of adults. During this time, maternal antibodies constitute a significant fraction of a baby's humoral immune system and thus, the neonatal period is a time when the immunological identity of an individual is not fully self-determined but is defined rather more in terms of 'mother'. In this same period, psychological development has been suggested to be undergoing a phase of the separation-individuation process when self-image is perceived in the context of maternal image.[23] The somatopsychic self-determination hypothesis interprets these two phenomena simply as explicit manifestations of whole system intent. Moreover, because of the importance of the early years for somatopsychic selfdevelopment, psychological disruptions or distortions during this time may have a significant impact on longer-temm immunological development. The observation that premature separation of rat pups from their mothers 15 days postnatally produced decreased immunological responsiveness at 40 days of age[24] may well be an example of this.

At other stages of life, different patterns of psychoimmune co-development will assume importance. At all ages immune responses contribute to and are affected by conscious and unconscious psychophysiological states and phenomena and so must be factors of the overall encoding for memory, learning and behaviour information. The observation that some people with Multiple Personality Disorder exhibit allergic symptoms when in certain personalities but not others[25] could be considered to be an illustration of this. Another example might be the modulating effects of aging on stress-associated immunological changes[26,27] which could be understood in terms of a progressive constraint or damping of response patterns as the 'selfimage' gradually becomes more established.

Self-tolerance viewed from a somatic perspective is an education process through which the immune system dynamically and recursively defines its own makeup and molecular identity.[1,28] Although this is a continual process throughout the life of an individual, it is most extensive early in life as discussed above. During such times of relative 'immunological immaturity' the immune system is generally regarded as being more susceptible to tolerance induction than at other times. This phenomenon can be interpreted within a self-determination framework as an indication of the general somatopsychic malleability during establishment of self-image at a time when the boundaries around what is later to be considered 'self' are less well-defined. An important implication of this sort of understanding is the possibility that gross manipulation of immune parameters during the early developmental phase of life (for example by extensive neonatal immunisation) may have the potential for more profound impact on psychoimmune self-development than comparable manipulations later in life.

VI. CONSEQUENCES FOR IMMUNOLOGY, HEALTH AND DISEASE

Within a somatopsychic self-determination model, similarities or parallels among contributing systems are deemed to arise out of the fundamental qualities of psychoneuroimmune wholeness and should be expressed in these terms rather than the more familiar language of cellular and molecular mechanisms. The evolution of our hypothesis into a coherent theory of somatopsychic self-determination will therefore require the development of a novel language that bridges and goes beyond that of the individual disciplines currently comprising psychoneuroimmunology. It will require a language built perhaps on the informational, semiotic and symbolic rather than purely mechanistic nature of the interactions occurring within an organism.[29-31] The relationship and limited interconvertibility between the analytic language of molecular mechanism and the more 'synthetic' language required for PNI phenomena can be illustrated by analogy with the languages of music. Music can be analysed sonically in terms of sound frequencies, intensities, durations and interval relationships. At a more integrated level it can be approached through a distinct language and syntax built out of the phenomena of harmony, counterpoint, polyphony, rhythm, motifs, themes. Information conveyed through this latter language (e.g., a structural coherence which gives a piece of music its particular character) can be explained but not adequately expressed in sonic terminology. Something similar to the language of music will be required to express a coherent theory for PNI.

An important consequence of our hypothesis is the necessity for a revised perspective on the influence of psychological and other processes on immune responses. If the immune system is as inextricably entwined with the psychophysiological self as we suggest, then associations between psychological and immunological variables must be understood as mutually generative dimensions of a greater whole. While explanation of isolated immunological events in cellular and/or molecular terms may be sufficient to understand their roles in immunity in the traditional sense, such explanation does not constitute understanding in the context of the psychoimmunological process. The concept of immune responsiveness to stimuli leading to the activation of effector mechanisms could be replaced by something akin to 'state-dependent receptiveness' to signals or events registered in a psychoimmune environment. By the very nature of the psychoimmune system, immunological components removed from the somatopsychic milieu and studied in isolation cannot necessarily be expected to behave in a way that faithfully models their behaviour *in situ*. While this does not invalidate scientific exploration of the molecular mechanics of specific immunological pathways, it does advise caution when extrapolating to immune behaviour *in vivo*. Perhaps most importantly it encourages an awareness of the limitations of animal models for human immunology and disease because of their fundamental inability to incorporate subjective human experience into their immunological framework. Focussing on the defensive and protective facets of immunological relationships to disease at the expense of psychophysiological aspects may mask potentially important clues to therapeutic and preventative interventions. Disease-associated immunological changes not only depend on the nature of any 'pathogenic' stimulus and the 'classical' immune response to it, but are expressions of the current dynamic state of the whole psychoneuroimmunedetermined self. As a result, psychoimmune (rather than immune) factors should be paramount considerations for understanding and treating any clinical illness.

Finally, to embrace a somatopsychic self-determination model as a basis for understanding immunological phenomena requires also that health and disease be understood from the same perspective. If health is considered to depend on the maintenance of optimal connectedness or coherence within and among all levels of a person (see figure 2), then immune responses are mechanisms for facilitating this process and supporting the integrity of the person in optimal relationship to his or her environment. Disease is consequently promoted by disconnection or separation and provides information about the dynamic process of somatopsychic existence. It therefore offers opportunities for organismic adaptive, evolutionary and/or transformative events in which the immune system is an integral participant. From the point of view of research and experimentation, the challenge is not only to identify and characterise critical associations between immunolodcal, psychological and other variables but to integrate them into a coherent theoretical framework. This will require the development of models along the lines proposed here, together with a language in which ideas can be rigorously expressed and questions framed in a psychoimmune context.

VII. REFERENCES

1. Vaz, N.M. and Varela, F.J., Self and non-sense: An organism-centred approach to immunology, *Med.Hypoth.*, 4, 231, 1978.
2. Jerne, N.K., , *Ann.Immunol.(Inst.Pasteur)*, 125C, 373, 1974.
3. Cohn, M., Nucleic Acids in Immunology, in , Plescia, I.J. and Brown, W., Eds., Springer-Verlag, Berlin, 1968, 671.
4. Zinkernagel, R.M. and Doherty, P.C., , *Ann.Immunol.(Inst.Pasteur)*, 125C, 373, 1974.
5. Pert, C.B., Ruff, M.R., Weber, R.J. and Herkenham, M., Neuropeptides and their receptors: A psychosomatic network, *J.Immunol.*, 135, 820s, 1985.
6. Weigent, D.A. and Blalock, J.E., Interactions between the neuroendocrine and immune systems: Common hormones and receptors, *Immunol.Rev.*, 188, 79, 1987.
7. Morley, J.E., Kay, N.E., Solomon, G.F. and Plotnikoff, N.P., Neuropeptides: Conductors of the immune orchestra, *Life.Sci.*, 41, 527, 1987.
8. Camara, E.G. and Danao, T.C., The brain and the immune system: A psychosomatic network, *Psychosomatics*, 30, 140, 1989.
9. Solomon, G.F., Psychoneuroimmunology: Interactions between central nervous system and immune system, *J.Neurosci.Res.*, 18, 1, 1987.
10. Khansari, D.N., Murgo, A.J. and Faith, R.E., Effects of stress on the immune system, *Immunol.Today*, 11, 170, 1990.
11. Booth, R.J., The psychoneuroimmune network: Expanding our understanding of immunity and disease, *NZ Med.J.*, 103, 314, 1990.
12. Kiecolt-Glaser, J.K. and Glaser, R., Psychological influences on immunity, *Psychosomatics*, 27, 621, 1986.
13. Cunningham, A.J., Mind, body and immune system, in *Psychoneuroimmunology*, Ader, R., Ed., Academic Press, 1981, 609.
14. Engel, B.T., Immune behavior, *Behav.Brain Sci.*, 8, 399, 1985.
15. Blalock, J.E., The immune system as a sensory organ, *J.Immunol.*, 132, 1067, 1984.
16. Blalock, J.E. and Smith, E.M., The immune system: Our mobile brain? *Immunol.Today*, 6, 115, 1985.
17. Burgio, G.R. and Martini, A., The individuality of the immune response, *Scand.J.Rheumatol.*, 66, 5s, 1987.

18. Payan, D.G., McGillis, J.P. and Goetzl, E.J., Neuroimmunology, *Adv.Immunol.*, 39, 299, 1986.

19. Besedovsky, H.O. and Sorkin, E., Network of immune-neuroendocrine interactions, *Clin.Exp.Immunol.*, 27, 1, 1977.

20. Singh, P.B., Brown, R.E. and Roser, B., Class I transplantation antigens in solution in body fluids and in the urine. Individuality signals to the environment, *J.exp.Med.*, 168, 195, 1988.

21. Brown, R.E., Roser, B. and Singh, P.B., Class I and class II regions of MHC both contribute to individual odors in congenic inbred strains of rats, *Behav.Genet.*, 19, 659, 1989.

22. Martin, J.B. and Reichlin, S., *Clinical Neuroendocrinology*, 2nd ed., F.A.Davis Co., Philadelphia, 1987, 672.

23. Mahler, M.S., Pine, F. and Bergman, A., *The Psychological Birth of the Human Infant*, Hutchinson & Co., Great Britain, 1975,

24. Ackerman, S.H., Keller, S.E., Schleifer, S.J., Shindledecker, R.D., Camerino, M., Hofer, M.A., Weiner, H. and Stein, M., Premature maternal separation and lymphocyte function, *Brain Behav.Immun.*, 2, 161, 1988.

25. Braun, B.G., Psychophysiologic phenomena in multiple personality and hypnosis, *Am.J.Clin.Hypnosis*, 26, 124, 1983.

26. Odio, M., Brodish, A. and Ricardo, M.J., Effects on immune responses by chronic stress are modulated by aging, *Brain Behav Immun*, 1, 204, 1987.

27. Naliboff, B.D., Benton, D., Solomon, G.F., Morley, J.E., Fahey, J.L., Bloom, E.T., Makinodan, T. and Gilmore, S.L., Immunological changes in young and old subjects during brief laboratory stress, *Psychosom.Med.*, 1990.(In Press)

28. Coutinho, A. and Bandeira, A., Tolerise one, tolerise them all: Tolerance is self-assertion, *Immunol.Today*, 10, 264, 1989.

29. Moerman, D.E., Anthropology of symbolic healing, *Curr.Anthropol.*, 20, 59, 1979.

30. Foss, L. and Rothenberg, K., *The Second Medical Revolution: From Biomedicine to Infomedicine*, Shambhala Press, Boston, 1988,

31. Cunningham, A.J., Information and health in many levels of man. Toward a more comprehensive theory of health and disease, *Advances*, 2, 32, 1986.

THE LINK BETWEEN IMMUNE RESPONSES AND BEHAVIOUR IN SHEEP

G.R. Gates[a], L.R. Fell[b], J.J. Lynch[c], D.B. Adams[d], J.P. Barnett[a], G.N. Hinch[e],
R.K. Munro[f] and H.I. Davies[g]

[a]Department of Psychology, University of New England, Armidale, 2351; [b]NSW Department
of Agriculture and Fisheries, Elizabeth Macarthur Agricultural Institute, Camden, 2570;
[c]CSIRO Divison of Animal Production, Pastoral Research Laboratory, Armidale, 2350;
[d]Bureau of Rural Resources, Department of Primary Industries and Energy, Canberra, ACT,
2600; [e]Department of Animal Science, [f]Department of Physiology and [g]Deparment of
Mathematics and Computing Science, University of New England, Armidale, 2351. Australia.

I. INTRODUCTION

Research findings from many quarters now indicate that central nervous system
processes influence immune system responses.[1] Behavioural conditioning as well as "natural"
experiments involving humans in stressful circumstances show that immunity can be enhanced
or suppressed and that these effects appear to be mediated by the neuroendocrine system.[2-4]
Research evidence also shows that the immune system *per se* influences neural and endocrine
function with consequent effects on behaviour. Parasites can modify the behaviour of their
hosts either through direct effects of burden or indirectly through changes to the immune
system. There is even evidence suggesting that behaviour is altered in such a way as to
increase the probability of parasite transmission.[5] In other words, the behaviour of the
infected host is altered in such a way that the host has an increased chance of passing on the
parasite to an uninfected conspecific.

The two-way interactions between nervous, endocrine and immune systems are not
yet well understood although there is promise that the relationships will be complex and
somewhat demanding to untangle (see Greenberg, Brown, Li & Dyck - this volume). It is
certainly the case that the endogenous opiates as well as a variety of neurohumours play a role
in these changes.[6,7]

One area of immune-behaviour change which appears to have received little attention
is the area of immune system challenge in organisms which have a standing or existing
immunity to an agent. Intuitively, one might think that once an animal has a well-established
immune response to an agent, that subsequent exposures to the agent might have a significant
and direct impact on the remobilization of immune defenses but little effect on behaviour.
However, from an evolutionary perspective there may be an advantage in both an immune
response as well as a behavioural response mediated by the immune-nervous system
interaction. In some cases the advantage may be to the host whereas in others, the parasite
may benefit.

In a 1989 paper, Fell and Shutt[8] described behavioural and physiological responses of sheep to acute surgical stress. Six to seven month old Merino wethers had wool and skin surgically removed from their perineal area (mulesing) in order to prevent "fly strike" (fly strike is a problem causing much debilitation and even deaths in Australian sheep flocks). The effects of mulesing included elevation of plasma cortisol and β-endorphin. In addition, the animals showed a marked aversion, in an arena test, to the human handlers who had held the sheep during the operation. Observations made of the animals over a 10 minute period by a hidden observer showed that the sheep stood further away from the handler in a 14 by 4 metre yard than from humans who did not take part in the surgery. Moreover, the sheep roamed less around the arena yard. Both effects lasted for more than five weeks. Fell and Shutt[8] concluded that the altered behaviour in the mulesed sheep was a "cognitive response to the stress associated with mulesing" (p. 292). In a subsequent study. Fell and colleagues[9] showed that Merino ewes which were given a serial immune challenge with the gastric nematode parasite *Haemonchus contortus* showed a significant reduction in the distance they stood from a human in the same arena test that was used for the first experiment. In addition, the animals which had been penned during the immune challenge displayed twice as much locomotor activity as sheep which had been left in an open paddock. They concluded that the arena test with small groups of sheep" may be a sensitive indicator of changes in complex behaviour" and may have predictive value concerning subsequent immune or stress responses. More importantly, their study seems to have been the first in large animals to report measurable behavioural change following immune system challenge in animals in which there was a high degree of immunity.

In the present paper we will describe a series of experiments which were designed to examine the impact of immune system challenge on behaviour of sheep with a well-established immune response to the parasite *Haemonchus contortus*. In addition, we report on experiments designed to identify some of the biochemical mediators which may be governing the behaviour changes seen in experimental sheep.

II. GENERAL METHOD

In the following section, the methods used in the experiments reported here are described in some detail.

A. EXPERIMENTAL ANIMALS
The animals used were Merino sheep which had been raised and maintained on a good quality pasture at CSIRO, "Chiswick" Pastoral Research Station, Armidale.

B. THE ARENA TEST
Arena testing was carried out in a covered, enclosed 13 by 3 metre yard with cement floor marked off into 1m grids (see Figure 1). The arena was very similar to that used by Fell and colleagues in their experiments (see Introduction). The grids were numbered from 1 to 39 and could be seen by observers placed directly above the grid floor on an elevated platform out of sight of the sheep. The arena was screened off with opaque 900mm high green shadecloth on three sides. At the eastern end where there was no shadecloth, a human, who had not taken part in the experimental manipulation of the sheep, stood motionless throughout each experimental condition. A group of eight sheep was placed in a 3m by 2m adjacent holding pen behind the human in full view of the experimental animals in the arena.

Four experimental animals at a time were let into the arena and left to travel around the arena at will. In most experiments, there were four groups of four sheep per treatment. Each sheep's position was recorded into a Toshiba lab-top computer every fifteen seconds by observers located on the elevated platform 2.5 metres above the arena floor. For most experiments forty observations were obtained, using an instantaneous time-sampling technique.[10]

Four behavioural measures were calculated for each experiment in the arena test:

1.   Distance (metres). The distance of animals from the human was recorded every fifteen seconds. For most experiments, average distance from the human over the 40 observation period is reported.

2.   Travel (in metres) over the 40 observations.

3.   Moves. The number of intergrid moves made by the animals in the arena over 40 observations.

4.   Spread (metres). Mean distance between the four animals at each observation which was then averaged over the 40 observations.

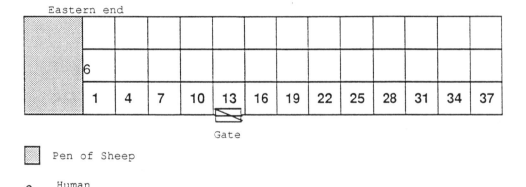

Figure 1. Plan of test arena. See text for full description of each experimental group.

As indicated previously, Fell and colleagues employed an arena test to measure behaviour change in sheep following immune system challenge and following mulesing. They found the test to be sensitive to these manipulations. However, their research did not get at the problem of what the test was actually measuring. The arena tests appears to produce a conflict of "drives" in sheep and in many ways resembles a classical approach/avoidance conflict.[11] The design of the arena is such that the test animals in the arena can see a larger group of eight sheep in the adjoining holding pen behind the human. Because Merinos have such a strong flocking "instinct", it is assumed that the experimental animals would have a

HAHNEMANN UNIVERSITY LIBRARY

strong tendency to approach the adjacent group of penned sheep. However, situated between the two groups of animals is a human. As sheep appear to have a natural aversion to humans,[12] it is presumed that the positioning of the human between the two groups of sheep leads to a conflict of drives. On the one hand, the experimental animals strive to avoid the human, while on the other the animals strive to approach their conspecifics. The conflict which is set up resembles the classical conflict seen in hungry rats approaching a known food source across a graded electric grid.

C. MANIPULATION OF THE IMMUNE RESPONSE

Animals involved in experiments with immune system challenge were required to have an established immunity. This was achieved by giving an oral infection of 10,000 *Haemonchus contortus* infective larvae four weeks prior to arena testing. Larvae were given with a drenching gun. This treatment ensured that all animals had a similar immune system status; that is, an acquired immunity to this gastric nematode popularly known as Barber's Pole Worm. Faecal samples were taken from the animals and results of faecal egg counts revealed that the animals had approximately 200 eggs per gram, indicating that a strong acquired immunity was established in all animals. Six and three days prior to arena testing, those animals which were to be included in an immune system challenge group received a further oral dose of 750 larvae in order to "challenge" their immunity. Doses given at these times are known to produce a reliable effect on behaviour (see Adams *et al*[13]). Other sheep were given an oral dose of water at the same times as the challenge groups.

The *Haemonchus contortus* larvae used in the experiments reported here were obtained from cultures of faeces of sheep harbouring a pure infection. Faecal egg counts were made by the McMaster method[14] on samples collected directly from the rectum.

D. EXPERIMENTAL PROCEDURE

All sheep had two numbers marked on their backs with scourable branding fluid; the first number indicated the experimental treatment to which the sheep belonged and the second indicated the order in which the sheep's positions in the arena test were to be recorded during testing. Sheep were allocated randomly to groups and position within groups. Animals were drafted and divided into their selected groups on the morning of arena testing and were penned in order of subsequent testing. Arena testing commenced at approximately 0900 h and was always completed by early afternoon. Testing was restricted to these times to avoid the possibility of confounding of results by diurnal variation in biochemistry. It is well known that a number of receptors for certain neurochemicals[15] and level of endogenous opiates vary as a function of time in the 24 hour circadian cycle (for discussion in relation to the immune system see chapter by Knapp elsewhere in this volume and Knapp, 1990[16]).

III. RESULTS

A. EXPERIMENT 1 - THE NATURE OF THE ARENA TEST

The aim of the first experiment was to establish whether the arena test produces an approach/avoidance conflict in sheep. In order to test this hypothesis, an experiment was designed to examine the behaviour of sheep in which the variables associated with the arena test were systematically altered. An experimental test was introduced where no human was present in the arena compound to determine whether the experimental sheep would approach

HAHNEMANN UNIVERSITY LIBRARY

the sheep in the adjacent pen. The outcome of this manipulation would indicate whether arena sheep were motivated to "join the flock" of the adjoining sheep. The same trial was then run with the human present but with and without the adjoining sheep present to determine whether the sheep found the human to be an aversive stimulus. In addition, trials were run with and without an opaque plastic in the fourth wall of the yard adjacent to the holding pen and with and without the human to determine whether being able to "see out" of the arena affected approach to this end of the arena. It was considered that the absence of shadecloth behind the human in previous experiments could have affected approach to the human even in the absence of adjoining sheep. Moreover, it was thought that the presence of the shadecloth would reduce the available visual cues and therefore reduce the drive of the experimental animals to approach conspecifics in the adjoining yard. In a sense, this shadecloth trial is a test of the potency of visual cues in the approach-avoidance conflict.

One hundred and twelve non pregnant Merino ewes were divided into seven experimental groups of sixteen animals each and were tested in the following order over two days:

Group	Experimental Condition
1	No adjoining sheep + human
2	No adjoining sheep + no human
3	Adjoining sheep + human
4	Adjoining sheep + no human
5	Shadecloth + no adjoining sheep + no human
6	Shadecloth + adjoining sheep + human
7	Shadecloth + adjoining sheep + no human

Four animals were tested at a time, Groups 1, 2 and 5 were tested first on both days to control for the possibility of arena sheep being able to detect olfactory cues from animals which had been previously housed in the adjacent pen. In the case of Groups 5 and 7 where no human was present, approach distance was the distance from the fence where the human had been standing for other experimental trials.

The behaviour of the animals was recorded and scored in the manner described in General Methods.

The means of the approach distances for the seven experimental manipulations are shown in Figure 2. The main findings of the experiment are that the animals which were tested in the presence of the human showed the greatest distance from the end of yard where the human stood. That is, the sheep tended to stand well away from animals in the adjoining yard when the human was present suggesting that the human was acting as an aversive stimulus to the arena animals.

In contrast, when the human was absent, the arena animals showed the greatest approach to the adjoining animals thus confirming that the adjoining animals act as a significant approach stimulus.

Analysis of travel data revealed that the least travel occurred in the three groups

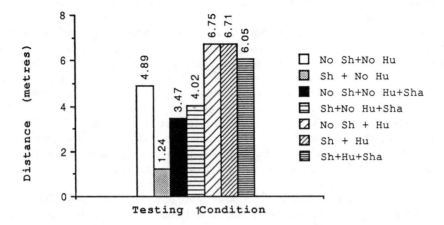

Figure 2.   Mean distance (in metres) from human for each group (n=16/group) of experimental sheep. See text for full description of each experimental group.

where the human was present (see Figure 3). The greatest travel occurred in the conditions where the shadecloth was present in all four walls of the arena but where the human was absent. The animals were notably agitated when all four walls were covered with shadecloth and there was no human focus for their apparent fear. The sheep appeared to attend to any sounds which came from outside the arena.

The least number of moves were made in the three conditions where the human was

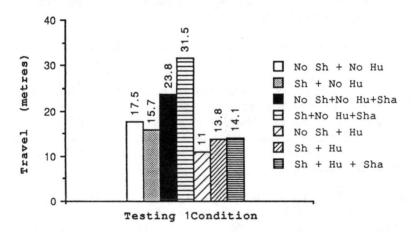

Figure 3.   Mean distance travelled by each group (n=16/group) of experimental animals. See text for full description of each experimental group.

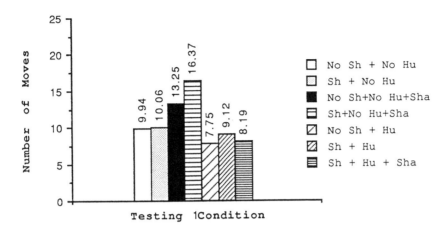

Figure 4. Mean number of moves made by each group (n=16/group) of experimental animals. See text for full description of each experimental group.

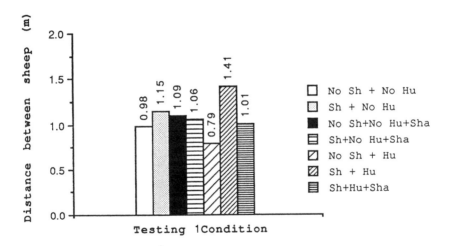

Figure 5. Distance between animals (spread) is shown for each experimental group (n=16/group). See text for full description of each experimental group.

present and the most in the condition where the shadecloth was present and the human absent (see Figure 4). Mean distances between animals in the 7 experimental conditions (see Figure 5) were not significantly different.

It is clear from this experiment that the presence of a human in the arena test acts as a noxious or aversive stimulus to the sheep. Similar responses were found by Fell and Shutt[8] in their experiment with mulesing. They also found an approach gradient in their experiment with the animals standing further away when they were exposed to the person who had been involved with the operation compared with the shorter distance from their normal handler. The current experiment did not examine the issue of approach gradient, but it is the case from the research of Fell and Shutt that the approach gradient can be manipulated experimentally. The arena test may be used as a device to test the noxious effects of animal husbandry practices on sheep and to test the impact of therapeutic or palliative interventions on such noxious effects. Testing also showed, very clearly, that the sheep in the arena test were strongly attracted to their counterparts in the adjoining pen. This attraction was dampened by the presence of the human being.

One other finding to emerge from the experiment is that not only is there an approach/avoidance conflict involved in the arena test, but there is also an effect on the motor behaviour of the animals in the arena. The motor or travelling behaviour of the animals changed with experimental manipulation. There was a dramatic increase in the activity of the animals in the absence of a focus for fear and in the absence of visual information about conspecifics in the adjacent pen. The travel data and distance data suggest that there may be two separate systems involved in the regulation of the behaviour of the animals in the arena test. Further research is needed to ascertain the factors which govern their functioning.

Overall, the evidence obtained in the present experiment shows that the arena test is a classic approach avoidance conflict.

B. EXPERIMENT 2 - ROLE OF ENDOGENOUS OPIATES: NALOXONE TEST

Fell and colleagues[9] found that sheep which had received a challenge dose of the gastric nematode *Haemonchus contortus* stood closer to the human in the arena test than non-challenged animals. The results suggested that the altered behaviour was due to acquired immunity to the worm rather than the worm *per se*, since an experiment involving oral infection with *H. contortus* administered to non-immune sheep produced no effect on approach distance in the non-immune animals compared to uninfected controls.

What then are the mechanisms which appear to be mediating the change in the behaviour of the challenged sheep? Recent research has revealed that there are opiate receptors located on various cells of the immune system[17] and that the endogenous opioids play a role in the modulation of elements of the immune system (see Plotnikoff and Miller, 1983[18]). The endogenous opioids are also known to play a major behavioural role in modulating "motivated" behaviour.[19] Since there are two-way interactions between the immune, endocrine and nervous systems, it was considered that the opiate peptides may be responsible for the closer approach behaviour to the human shown by the immune-challenged sheep. The hypothesis that opiates were involved in the immune-challenge response was examined by Barnett et al.[20] who administered the opiate buprenorphine to uninfected sheep and found that the drug-treated animals showed closer approach behaviour to the human in the arena test than those injected with saline. This result was similar to that seen in sheep receiving a challenge infection of *H. contortus*. To further test the hypothesis that the endogenous opiates are involved in closer approach behaviour, immunologically challenged and unchallenged animals were given the opiate antagonist naloxone. It was predicted that those animals given naloxone would stand further away from the human as they would no longer be behaviourally "protected" by endogenous opiates.

Four groups of 16 animals were used in this experiment. Two groups received immunological challenge with *H. contortus* as described in General Methods and two groups were left unchallenged. The four groups were as follows in terms of experimental treatment:

1. Unchallenged, no drug
2. Challenged. no drug
3. Unchallenged, naloxone
4. Challenged, naloxone

Fifteen minutes prior to arena testing, the naloxone treated animals were given a 0.8mg dose of naloxone by intravenous injection into the jugular vein. Sheep were tested in the arena test in the manner described in the General Methods section.

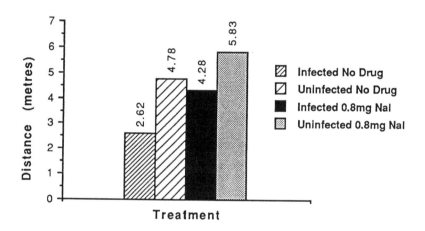

Figure 6. Mean distance (in metres) from human sheep stood for each experimental condition (n = 16/group). See text for full description of each experimental group.

Figure 6 shows the results of arena testing. Those animals who had been challenged with a trickle infection of *H. contortus* stood significantly closer to the human than those who remained unchallenged. In addition, those animals who were treated with naloxone stood significantly further away whether they had been challenged with *H. contortus* or not.

The results of this experiment and that of Barnett et al.[20] suggest that the endogenous opiates are involved in the changed approach behaviour of immunologically-challenged sheep in the arena test. While the use of an opiate antagonist is not a comprehensive test of an endogenous opiate mechanism,[21] it is at least an additional piece of evidence which supports such a hypothesis.

C. EXPERIMENT 3 - MIMICKING OF ARENA TEST BEHAVIOUR WITH OPIATES

The previous experiment, along with the earlier work of Barnett et al.[20] with single dose buprenorphine, suggested that endogenous opiates play a role in immune-challenge behaviour change. However, what was not clear from the single dose buprenorphine study was whether or not the behaviour change seen was dose dependent. If endogenous opiates are modulating the distance the sheep are from the human, then it might be expected that different doses might affect the distance that the sheep stand from the human. In the following experiment sheep were given five different doses of buprenorphine.

Seven groups of immunologically unchallenged wethers were used in this experiment. The groups were:

1. Nil treatment
2. Physiological saline control
3. 0.5ml buprenorphine (0.003mg/kg)
4. 0.75ml buprenorphine (0.005mg/kg)
5. 1.0ml buprenorphine (0.007mg/kg)
6. 1.5ml buprenorphine (0.01 mg/kg)
7. 2.0ml buprenorphine (0.01 mg/kg)

The saline control was introduced to control for the effects of injection. As for the previous experiment, the animals were given the drugs and saline by intravenous jugular injection and the methods for recording and observation of behaviour were the same as those described in the General Methods section. The buprenorphine (Temgesic R, Reckitt and Colman) and saline were given fifteen minutes before arena testing.

The results of the experiment are shown in Figure 7. Buprenorphine at all doses resulted in the animals being closer to the human in the arena test compared to controls; however, the distance effect was non-linear in nature. The reason for this non-linearity is not clear and requires further exploration.

An unexpected finding of the study was that saline injection *per se* has a significant effect on distance of approach, there being no difference between the saline and second highest dose group of buprenorphine in approach distance. The reason for this effect is also not clear. It is possible that the 2ml injection of sodium chloride is having some direct effect on behaviour. This explanation is unlikely. A more likely reason for the injection effect is that the procedure for capturing the animal for injection, combined with holding and injection into the jugular vein may be stressful to the animals and induce an increase in endogenous opiates or other stress-related substances. The act of taking blood samples is known to cause ACTH release.[22] Routine handling procedures, including up-ending, affect cortisol and glucose levels.[23,24] Such mechanisms may help to explain the closer approach of saline-injected animals to the human. Further experimentation is required to elucidate this mechanism.

One final interesting observation from this study was that at higher doses of buprenorphine, some of the animals approached and came into contact with the human in the arena test. Some of these animals pushed themselves between the fence of the adjoining pen and the human's legs and

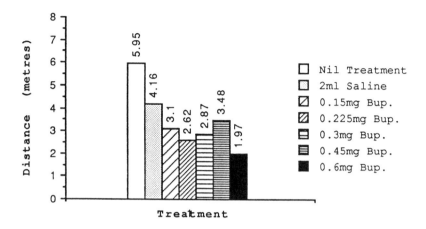

Figure 7. Distance (in metres) sheep stood from human in the arena test by experimental groups (n=16/group). See text for full description of each experimental group.

showed no outward signs of fear. In addition, some of the animals exhibited non-nutritive eating behaviour, chewing movements, mounting behaviour, agitation and aggression. Such behaviours resembled the stereotypical responses that are seen in animals kept in sensory-deprived environments and in situations of high unpredictability.[22] Dantzer[25] reports that administration of opiates produces hyperactivity and stereotypy and Cooper *et al*[26] have evidence that endogenous opioid peptides are involved in ingestive behaviour.

D. EXPERIMENT 4 - EFFECTS OF OPIATES ON FLOCK BEHAVIOUR AND STRUCTURE

Immune system challenge may not only have implications for physiological changes within an animal but may also produce behaviour changes which have significance for survival or for spread of a disease. Infection of mice with the nematode parasite *Trichinella spiralis* changed their social dominance and interactions with other mice.[27] It was suggested that loss of social status might lead to increased vulnerability of infected animals to predation and ultimately to parasitic transmission to a second animal. Such a finding supports the notion of parasitic manipulation of host behaviour.[5]

The present experiment was undertaken to better understand the dynamics of the flocking behaviour of sheep in the arena test. Particular attention was given to the effect that the exogenously administered opiates might have on the behaviour of groups of four sheep when varying numbers of animals were given this pharmacological agent. It was considered that exogenous opiate administration to 1, 2, 3 or 4 sheep within the group of four was much less complicated and time-consuming than administration of a larval challenge to a variable number of animals over the time frame required for immune system challenge with the parasite *H. contortus*.

Animals were randomly assigned to one of six treatments and their behaviour was recorded over 80 observations rather than the usual forty to make sure that adequate time was available to observe flock dynamics. The six groups of sixteen animals were as follows:

Day	Group	Treatment
1	1	Nil treatment
	2	1 sheep 0.225mg (0.005mg/kg) buprenorphine + 3 sheep 0.75ml saline
2	3	4 sheep 0.75ml saline
	4	4 sheep 0.225mg (0.005mg/kg) buprenorphine
3	5	3 sheep 0.225mg (0.005mg/kg) buprenorphine + 1 sheep 0.75ml saline
	6	2 sheep 0.225mg (0.005mg/kg) buprenorphine + 2 sheep 0.75ml saline

Fifteen minutes prior to arena testing, all groups, except the nil treatment group, received either 0.005mg/kg of buprenorphine or normal saline by intravenous injection into the jugular vein.

The summary results for the 80 observations for the six groups are shown in Figure 8. As for "40" observation experiments, the four saline treatment sheep kept the greatest distance from the human and the four buprenorphine group, the closest approach distance. Apart from the 2 buprenorphine-treated animals (group 6), there was a stepwise progression from greatest to least approach distance by the opiate-treated animals, according to the number of animals receiving the opiate.

Time series analysis of these data indicates that treatment with an opiate produces different surges of movement to that seen in control animals but the time sampling methodology used for data collection does not permit further analysis.

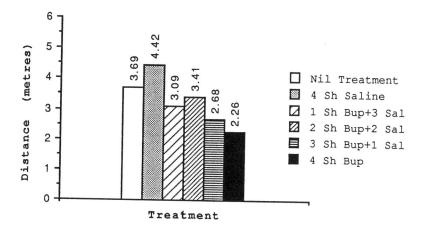

Figure 8. Mean distance (in metres) for 80 observations for each experimental group (n=16/group). See text for full description of each experimental group.

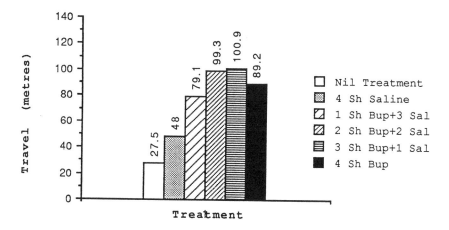

Figure 9. Mean travel distance for 80 observations for each experimental group (n=16/group). See text for full description of each experimental group.

The results of the present experiment show that opiate manipulation has an effect on the flocking and approach behaviour of sheep. In contrast to the findings from Rau and Putter's study,[27] where infected animals appeared less dominant, the opiate-treated animals of the present study showed altered social behaviour, but no signs of subordination. Opiate-treated animals were particularly dominant and aggressive toward other members of the group of sheep in the arena. The reasons for the differences are not clear and certainly many possibilities may be canvassed. Unfortunately, there is no comparable work in large animals for purposes of comparison.

As in previous opiate experiments, the opiate-treated animals showed stereotypical and agitated behaviour. In addition, the opiates appear to interfere with the sheep's natural avoidance of humans in the arena test and produce an increase in locomotory behaviour. The findings also suggest that the opiates interfere with the animals natural flocking behaviour as the treated animals tended to abandon the other members of their group to move toward the animals in the adjoining pen. The findings of this study therefore support the notion that opiates degrade flocking behaviour.

The question of whether sheep which have been challenged with *H. contortus* would also show a change in flocking behaviour remains unanswered but clearly the results of the

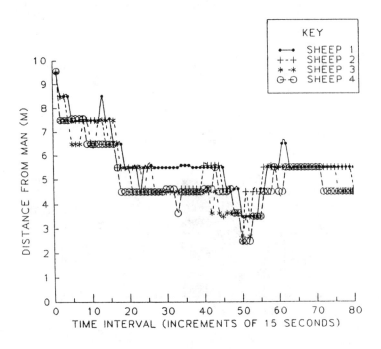

Figure 10. Distance that each sheep (n=4) stood from human over 80 observations. None of the animals received drug treatments.

present experiment encourage further experimentation. Such an experiment should involve data collection in real time so that account may be taken of the factors which govern the initiation and termination of behavioural sequences.

Analysis of the mean distances travelled by the 6 groups (see Figure 9) is far more revealing of the impact of buprenorphine on the behaviour of the animals than distance from the human. The least travel was shown by the nil treatment groups and the most by the buprenorphine-treated animals. Saline showed significantly more travel than nil-treatment animals, but significantly less than opioid treated sheep. The number of sheep treated with buprenorphine had an influence on travel distance.

Mean number of moves mirrored travel data but the mean distance or spread data was less clear cut with only the nil treatment and 2 sheep buprenorphine animals being signifcantly different from the remainder.

Representation of the data in the form shown in Figure 10 and 11 allow the reader to see that the dynamics of the behaviour of sheep with different treatments are far more complex than summary data indicate. These Figures show the behaviour of two groups of four sheep from the six different treatment conditions over the eighty observations of the current

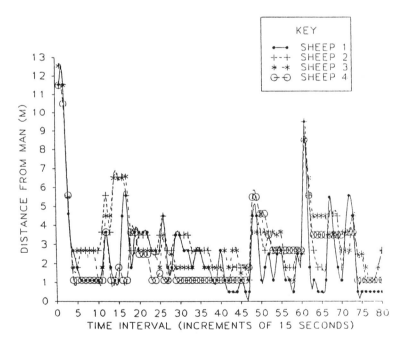

Figure 11. Distance that each sheep (n=4) stood from human over 80 observations. The first sheep received a 0.005 mg/kg i.v. dose of buprenorphine.

experiment. Figure 10 shows the behaviour of four animals from the nil treatment group. In contrast to other experimental groups, the animals in the nil treatment condition tended to remain stationary during the last ten minutes of the 20 minute observation period. Straight horizontal lines in Figure 10 indicate when the animals are stationary. Figure 11 represents the behaviour of one group of animals in the 1 sheep opiate condition. In contrast to the nil treatment group, these animals displayed markedly increased locomotory behaviour as well as closer approach to the human during testing. Similar results are shown for the other opiate groups.

IV. GENERAL DISCUSSION

This is the first time, to our knowledge, that the impact of immune challenge on the behaviour of immunologically-primed animals has been studied in any detail in large animals. The original work of Fell et al[9] showed that when immune sheep were given trickle reinfection with the nematode *H. contortus* their behaviour changed in an arena test. The reason for the change was not apparent and linle was known concerning the nature of the arena test. Subsequent investigations, reported here and elsewhere (see Barnett et al.[20]) suggest that the endogenous opiates may play a role in the behaviour change. The opiate antagonist, Naloxone was shown to modify behaviour of immune challenged sheep but not sheep without immunity. In addition, the administration of the opioid buprenorphine brought about changes in behaviour similar to those seen following immune challenge in terms of approach distance, but the dose-response relationship was found to be non-linear. The mechanisms underlying this nonlinearity are not clear and warrant further investigation. Interestingly, opiate-administered groups walked significantly more than controls whereas those challenged with *H. contortus* travelled signiflcantly less. The reason for this finding is also not clear and further investigation with other opiates which affect different opiate receptors in the brain is warranted. In addition, the endogenous opiate and related chemical changes which occur following immune challenge should be studied. This may give some clue as to the classes of substances which govern the behaviour change. The fact that an exogenously administered opioid has the same effect as immune challenge for one segment of behaviour (approach distance), but quite the opposite effect for another (locomotory behaviour) suggests that at least two separate neurobehavioural systems are involved in the effects of immune challenge. We are currently investigating this possibility with other pharmacological agents.

The experiments reported here also indicate that the arena test resembles a classic approach-avoidance conflict and is a sensitive measure of sheep behaviour. Fell and Shut[8] showed that surgical treatment of sheep led to behaviour changes in terms of approach distance. The current experiments show that the sheep handling and injection of sheep produces significant change in approach distance. In view of the sensitivity of the arena test to such varying procedures, it may well be a very simple and practical test for examining the impact on sheep of a variety of animal husbandry practices and for testing for the effects of various pharmacological agents and vaccines.

One serendipitous finding to emerge from the experiments reported here relates to the multiplicity of effects of the endogenous opiates on the behaviour of the sheep. Stereotypic behaviours such as biting and chewing were very clearly seen. It would appear that the experimental paradigm used here is a very useful one for investigating procedures that might be used to relieve or control the "bad habits" or stereotypies seen in intensive animal production.

The ecological significance of the behavioural changes seen in the sheep following immune system challenge is not clear. Whether the behaviour changes are epiphenomenal or of survival value to the individual or group or to the parasite itself warrants further investigation. It is the case that parasite burden *per se* alters the behaviour of horses and bighorn sheep and affects survival and reproductive success.[28,29] In mice, parasite burden influences parasite spread.[5] Whether or not immune challenge in immunologically-primed animals has similar effects or some quite separate function is not understood. If immune challenge does make the animals less fearful, then it is possible that they may become more susceptible to predation. Whether this has implications for parasite spread, or not, can be empirically tested.

The specific pathway by which challenge from a trickle infection of *H. contortus* brings about the changes in approach distance and locomotory behaviour in sheep is unclear. The endogenous opiates appear to be clearly implicated in the changes seen, but the steps by which the nematode exerts its effects remain to be identified. What is clear from the present experiments is that the relationship between the immune system and the central nervous system is a two-way process. It is well established in the literature that the central nervous system alters the immune system. The current experiments show that immune system challenge brings about changes in the central nervous system which are reflected in behaviour. The alterations are not the direct effects of acute systemic illness associated with parasite burden but rather are related to changes associated with immune system challenge *per se*.

V. REFERENCES

1. Riley, V., Psychoneuroendocrine influences on immunocompetence and neoplasia, *Science*, 212, 1100, 1981.
2. Ader, R. and Cohen, N., CNS-immune system interactions: Conditioning pehnomena, *Behav.Brain Sci.*, 8, 379, 1985.
3. Glaser, R., Rice, J., Speicher, C.E., Stout, J.C. and Kiecolt-Glaser, J.K., Stress depresses interferon production by leukocytes concomitant with a decrease in natural killer cell activity, *Behav.Neurosci.*, 100, 675, 1986.
4. Kelley, K.W., Cross-talk between the immune and endocrine systems, *J.Anim.Sci.*, 66, 2095, 1988.
5. Edwards, J.C., The effects of Trichinella spiralis infection on social interactions in mixed groups of infected and uninfected male mice, *Anim.Behav.*, 36, 529, 1988.
6. Frandsen, J.C., Parasites as stressors: Plasma cortisol responses of goats infected with the stomach worm Haemonchus contortus to exogenous corticotropin (ACTH), *Vet.Parasitol.*, 23, 43, 1987.
7. Kavaliers, M. and Podesta, R., Opioid involvement in parasite-induced behavioural modifications: Evidence from hamsters infected with Schistosoma mansoni,

Can.J.Zool., 66, 2653, 1988.

8.   Fell, L.R. and Shutt, D.A., Behavioural and hormonal responses to acute surgical stress in sheep, *Appl.Anim.Behav.Sci.*, 22, 283, 1989.

9.   Fell, L.R., Lynch, J.J., Adams, D.B., Hinch, G.N. and Munro, R.K., Behavioural and physiological effects in sheep of a stressful situation and an immunological challenge, unpublished data, 1990.

10.   Tyler, S., Time sampling: A matter of convention, *Animal Behavior*, 27, 801, 1979.

11.   Woodgush, D.G.M., *Elements of ethology*, Chapman and Hall, New York, 1983,

12.   Hutson, G.D., "Flight distance" in Merino sheep, *Anim.Prod.*, 35, 231, 1982.

13.   Adams, D.B., Fell, L.R., Lynch, J.J., Barnett, J.P., Gates, G.R. and Hinch, G.N., The time-course of behavioural effects of immune responses to challenge infection with Haemonchus contortus in sheep, unpublished data, 1990.

14.   Barger, I.A., Le Jambre, L.F., Georgie, J.R. and Davies, H.I., Regulation of Haemonchus contortuspopulations in sheep exposed to continuous infection, *Int.J.Parasit.*, 15, 529, 1985.

15.   Codd, E.E. and Byrne, W.L., Seasonal variation in the apparent number of naloxone binding sites, in *Endogenous and Exogenous Opiate Agonists and Antagonists. Proceedings of the International Narcotic Research Club Conference*, Way, E.L, Ed., Pergamon Press,Inc., Massachusetts,USA, 1980,

16.   Knapp, M.S., Computing for clinical chronobiology, for bibliography compilation and for data storage, graphical presentation and statistical analysis, in *Chronobiology: Its role in Clinical Medicine, General Biology, and Agriculture, Part B*, Wiley-Liss,Inc., 1990, 449.

17.   Mehrishi, J.N. and Mills, I.H., Opiate receptors on Lymphocytes and platelets in man, *Clin.Immunol.Immunopath.*, 27, 240, 1983.

18.   Plotnikoff, N.P. and Miller, G.C., Enkephalins as immunomodulators, *Int.J.Immunopharmacol.*, 5, 437, 1983.

19.   Faneslow, M.S., Calcagneni, D.J. and Helmstetter, F.J., Modulation of appetitively and adversively motivated behaviour by the Kappa opioid antagonist MR 2266, *Behav.Neurosci.*, 103, 663, 1989.

20.   Barnett, J.P., Fell, L.R., Lynch, J.J., Adams, D.B., Hinch, G.N., Munro, R.K. and Gates, G.R., Effect of opiate antagonist and antihistamine on behaviour of immune ewes infected with Haemonchus contortus. Proceedings of the 17th Annual Conference of the Australasian Society for the Study of Animal Behaviour. University of Queensland, Brisbane. April, 1990.

21.   Sawynok, J., Pinsky, C. and LaBella, F.S., Minireview on the specificity of naloxone as an opiate antagonist, *Life Sci.*, 25, 1621, 1979.

22.   Broom, D.M., *Biology of Behaviour: Mechanisms, Functions and Applications*, Cambridge University Press, New York, 1981,

23.   Hargreaves, A.L. and Hutson, G.D., The stress response in sheep during routine handling procedures, *Appl.Anim.Behav.Sci.*, 26, 83, 1990.

24.   Hargreaves, A.L. and Hutson, G.D., An evaluation of the contribution of isolations, up-ending and wool removal to the stress response to shearing, *Appl.Anim.Behav.Sci.*, 26, 103, 1190.

25.   Dantzer, R., Behavioural,physiological and functional aspects of stereotyped behaviour. A review and a re-interpretation, *J.Anim.Sci.*, 103, 663, 1986.

26.   Cooper, S.J., Jackson, A., Kirkham, T.C. and Turkish, S., Endorphins, opiates and food intake, in *Endorphins, opiates and behavioural processes*, Rodgers, R.J. and

Cooper, S.J., Eds., John Wiley, Chichester, 1987,

27.   Rau, M.E. and Putter, L., Running responses of Trichinella spiralis-infected CD-1 mice, *Parasitology*, 89, 579, 1984.

28.   Festa-Bianchet, M., Nursing behaviour of bighorn sheep: correlates of ewe age, parasitism, lamb age, birth date and sex, *Anim.Behav.*, 36, 1445, 1988.

29.   Rubenstein, D.I. and Hohmann, M.E., Parasites and social behaviour of island feral horses, *Olkos*, 55, 312, 1989.

PSYCHONEUROENDOCRINE CONCOMITANTS OF THE EMOTIONAL EXPERIENCE ASSOCIATED WITH RUNNING AND MEDITATION

Jane Harte

School of Behavioural Sciences,
James Cook University of North Queensland, Townsville. Australia

I. ABSTRACT

This paper examines the relationships between psychological and neuroendocrine variables in two metabolically bipolar types of action and experience: vigorous exercise (running) and meditation. A review of literature features the empirical work from our own laboratories, which is based on the notion that two metabolically different activites can lead to similar positive emotional changes because they are related to similar endocrine changes. It is also argued that a multi-levelled theory of emotion most adequately accounts for general emotional experience. Studies discussed include the effects of running and meditation on urinary adrenaline, noradrenaline and cortisol, as well as plasma 6-endorphin, corticotropic-releasing hormone (CRH) and cortisol. Overall, urinary noradrenaline and plasma CRH immunoreactivity were found to be elevated after both running and meditation. The implications of these findings are discussed in relation to the hypothalamic-pituitary-adrenocortical axis.

II. INTRODUCTION

A biological basis of behaviour is now considered to be axiomatic in many circles. Physiological psychology, unlike other areas in psychology, never really relinquished its origins in 19th century medicine, and is now legitimately reunited in the study of immunology and endocrinology. Attempts to separate "the mental" from "the physical" are outdated; instead, we illustrate the interplay between entities of what, in the end, is a biological organism surviving in a biological ecosystem. Further, we are now looking into the biologically adaptive responses associated with aversive conditions such as depression and anxiety, two of the emotional experiences associated with the general stress response.

There needs to be some clarification of the terms *stress* and *emotion*. The early idea that stress is a strain on an organism's homeostasis has developed into the study of physiological responses such as the *general adaptation syndrome*.[1] In questioning whether all stress is particularly aversive, Lazarus[2] distinguished between *eustress* - a positive, pleasant experience, and *dystress* - a negative, unpleasant one. There is some debate about the nature of emotions, but their association with visceral and physiological changes links them to stress responses. Emotions are the psychophysiological expressions of stress which, according to Cannon,[3] have survival value for the individual. Coping with stress, then, involves emotion.

In studying emotion, investigators are concerned with an individual's subjective rating of mood or affect, together with visceral and endocrine changes.

Much of the psychoneuroendocrine research on emotion has concerned pathological conditions with the premise that this data could be extrapolated to normal populations. An abnormal level of hormone X in clinical depression, for example, is thought to indicate a particular role for X, either by its elevation or attenuation, in maintaining homeostasis in normal cases. The work which is overviewed in this paper deals with what could be called supranormal cases. Two positive emotion-stimulating activities, running and meditation, were chosen for their anti-stressant effects and studied accordingly. This approach is propagated by the possibility that normal people may be trained to deal with stress by engaging in such pastimes. From a neuroendocrinological point of view, why these activities are anti-stressant and generate overall physiological and psychological adaptive responses provides for an interesting line of inquiry.

III. THEORETICAL CONSIDERATIONS

A. THE IMPLICATION OF PHYSIOLOGY IN EMOTION

Research conducted this century has successfully discounted the idea that emotion is merely a subjective evaluation. Early theories by James,[4] Calkins[5] and Meyer[6] importantly pointed to CNS activity as intrinsic in emotional experience, although other aspects of their respective theories were of little value. When Cannon[3] demonstrated that emotional behaviour involves the release of adrenaline from the adrenal medulla into the circulation together with peripheral responses, the way was paved for the study of neuroendocrine concomitants of emotion. Later, Frankenhaeuser's research showed that adrenaline and another catecholamine, noradrenaline, were released in response according to environmental and psychosocial stimuli, thus implicating the adrenal medulla in emotional responses (see Frankenhaeuser[7]). Selye[8] showed the link between emotional and adrenal-cortical activity after he noticed an enlargement of the adrenal cortex in animals exposed to stressful situations. Secretion of the principle hormone of the adrenal cortex, cortisol, has more recently been shown to be increased in humans exposed to a variety of psychosocial and physical stimuli such as aircraft flight, examinations and dental visits (see Smith)[9] or in response to uncertain or novel situations such as exposure to erotic or suspense films.[10]

A well tested, comprehensive, neuroanatomical map of emotional experience has not yet been found, although the limbic areas, cerebral cortex and brain stem appear to be implicated. Particular attention has been placed on the hypothalamus after Cannon and Bard demonstrated differences in emotional responses in animals whose brains were sectioned at various levels. Their conclusion was that the organization of the sequences of neuroanatomical responses in emotion are somehow organized in the hypothalamus.[11] Studies of the adjoining pituitary gland, and its role in both secreting hormones and regulating the secretion of hormones by other glands (such as the adrenal gland) began to put emphasis on inter-relating CNS subsystems in emotion (and other regulated behaviour), combining neuroanatomical and endocrine elements, and linking the hypothalamus to target glands. One such subsystem is referred to as the hypothalamic-pituitary-adrenocortical axis (HPA).

Adrenocorticotropic hormone (ACTH), procesesed from a larger precurser molecule, pro-opiomelaninocortin (POMC), and which is released by the anterior pituitary, appears to be a particularly important link in the responses of the HPA, and serves to stimulate the secretion of androgenic steroids from the adrenal cortex, amongst other corticoids.[12] The effects of ACTH are varied, but its release during anxiety points to a role in stress reduction; an idea supported by the observation of heightened positive emotions in patients receiving therapeutic doses of the hormone (see Cohen & Ross[13]). Other important findings imply that ACTH is involved in memory and learning,[14] and selective attention.[15]

With a refinement in measurement techniques such as radioimmunoassay, other HPA hormones have been implicated in emotion. The discovery of the endogenous opiates,

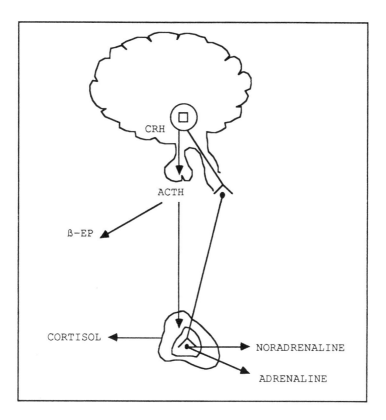

Figure 1 The hypothalamic-pituitary-adrenocortical axis. CRH from the hypothalamus stimulates the secretion of ACTH and β-EP through the anterior pituitary, which in turn elicits the release of cortisol from the adrenal cortex. CRH also acts on the adrenal medulla, resulting in adrenaline and noradrenaline secretion.

endorphins, in 1975 by Teschemacher and colleagues, and the isolation of the potent 6-endorphin (B-EP), which is released by the pituitary gland, prompted a new line of research in pain modulation, diuretic mediation, depression, addiction and stress. The search for a corticotrophic releasing hormone which stimulates the release of ACTH and 6-EP ended when such a compound was isolated in 1981 by Vale and colleagues, and ultimately labelled CRH. Attention then moved away from 6-EP to CRH as the more influential factor in emotional and other regulatory responses. Findings reviewed by Taylor and Fishman[16] indicate that abnormal CRH secretions occur in clinical depression, Cushings Syndrome and anorexia. The contemporary model of the HPA axis and the secretion of according hormones mentioned here is illustrated in Figure 1. Endocrine responses have so developed into a major area of study in the psychophysiology of emotion.

B. A HEURISTIC MODEL OF EMOTION

In reviewing the history of theoretical approaches to emotion, it is revealed that there is a complicated series of peripheral, endocrine and subjective responses involved. In order to most adequately understand the emotional experience, the approach to research should be multi-levelled. Staats and Eifert[17] argue that too many theories have been overly specific in that important variables such as personality, motivation and learning have been ignored in

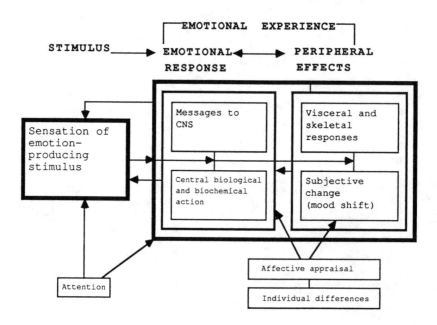

Figure 2 Conceptual model of the process of emotion, showing feedback loops and mediators.

favour of descriptions of one or a few aspects of the overall experience. With this in mind, the heuristic model illustrated in Figure 2 was developed by expanding on a basic stimulus-response relationship. It is assumed that the process of emotion is generally a linear phenomenon, from an original sensation to a final affective change. First, a stimulus is perceived, which percipitates an initial response involving the CNS and endocrine changes. Related to this response are peripheral effects, and the perception of affective change. Mediators in the process are attention, immediate appraisal and individual differences (such as personality and motivation). Further, when feedback loops are added, peripheral/subjective effects may influence emotional response. The entire emotional experience (response and peripheral/subjective effects) may influence the original sensation stage, providing that the stimulus is ongoing.

IV. EMPIRICAL FINDINGS

A. ENDOCRINE AND AFFECTIVE CONSEQUENCES OF RUNNING

Exercise is well documented as a mood enhancer. Barhke and Morgan,[18] Griest *et al*,[19] Kostrabula,[20] Morgan[21-23] and others, have written extensively on the affective beneficience (a term used by Morgan) of sports and exercise, especially with implications in treatment for depression. Further, the observation that athletes often feel elated after exercise may be considered one incentive for continuing with the activity. Apart from explanations involving state dependence (see Blaney[24]), this has contributed to the ensuing emphasis on the addictive quality of exercise.[25-27] Further, it is argued by Harte[28] that the study of sports provides for a good application of a multi-levelled theory of emotion. As running is one if the more common types of exercise studied, only this medium is discussed in what follows.

Running has been shown to increase catecholamine secretion in humans due to hypoglycaemia, dehydration, increased perceived exertion and rising body temperature.[29] Because of the link between adrenaline, noradrenaline and stress, these amines were implicated in the antidepressant effects of exercise.[30] We have found elevated affective change and urinary levels of adrenaline, noradrenaline and cortisol after athletes ran outdoors at training pace for 45 minutes (Harte & Eifert, unpublished data). Although we found no significant correlation between the hormones and mood change in the outdoor condition, when attention and environment were manipulated, an interesting trend was evident. The same subjects were required to tediously run on a treadmill for 45 minutes, with nothing to look at but a blank wall, and nothing to listen to but feedback of their own breathing. Not only did noradrenaline and cortisol excretions increase markedly, but they were significantly correlated with negative affective change. Apart from demonstrating an interplay between endocrine function, physical exertion, attention, environment and affect, this finding has applications in the design of training programs.[31]

Studies showing an increase in the secretion of plasma 6-endorphin during exercise are prolific (see Carr *et al*,[32] Colt *et al*,[33] Fraoli *et al*,[34] and Gambert *et al* [35]). When the opiate antagonist naloxone was used to block endorphin uptake, running associated mood shifts were observed to be attenuated[36-38] except when the dose of naloxone was comparatively small.[39] Such findings have therefore implicated 6-endorphin in the anti-depressant effects of exercise. In a recent study by Harte (unpublished data), plasma immunoreactive 6-endorphin and CRH were shown to increase after athletes ran for over an hour. Further, such HPA activity was significantly correlated with positive affective change. Surprisingly, plasma cortisol showed no significant change.

Remembering the contraints of the heuristic working model of emotion, CNS and HPA activity not only generate subjective and peripheral responses, but these responses in turn may effect the CNS and HPA, providing the stimulus is ongoing. In the case of running, this implies that altered mood state and peripheral change both affect and are affected by endocrine function. This seems straightforward, but the question that remains is, to what extent is it peripheral change (versus affective change) that affects endocrine function? Meditation, as a hypometabolic emotion-enhancing activity, provides for a good comparison to running. By eliminating hypermetabolic peripheral change, it may be possible to investigate more directly the link between affective change and endocrine function.

B. ENDOCRINE AND AFFECTIVE CONSEQUENCES OF MEDITATION

Although there is a great deal written about the peripheral and subjective effects of meditation, endocrine studies are rare, and those in the literature are generally poorly executed. There are, however, indications that during concentrative meditation (a term which includes Tanscendental and some types of Yogic Meditation), decreased adrenocortical activity occurs. Jevning *et al*[40] found decreased levels of plasma cortisol during Transcendental Meditation (TM) and in practitioners generally compared to nonpractitioners. Bujatti and Reidere[41] investigated catecholamine activity indirectly by measuring the metabolite vanillic-mandelic acid (VMA) in urine before and after subjects practised TM. The overall decrease in VMA was interpreted as decreased catecholamine activity. A similar approach was used by Udupa *et al*[42,43] but they found an increase in VMA after subjects practised Hatha Yoga. This type of yoga, unlike the more quiescent TM, is based on physical stimulation through breathing exercises and postures, and it is likely that the differing results were due to differences in meditation practice.

The variable attention was manipulated by Eifert and Harte (unpublished data) in a study of urinary cortisol, noradrenaline and adrenaline during concentrative meditation in regular practitioners. Two test conditions were compared to a control period. The first condition involved simple meditation and during the second, subjects were asked to meditate whilst listening to bland music. Adrenaline excretion showed no variation according to pre and post test measures and noradrenaline rose significantly after both conditions. Interesting was the finding that cortisol decreased during the first condition and increased during the taped music session. Cortisol also correlated significantly with negative affective change in the second condition. In summary, noradrenaline was linked to the affective arousal (positive and negative) associated with two types of quiescent activity, while positive affect was related to a decrease in cortisol and negative affect, to an increase in cortisol .

C. A COMPARISON OF RUNNING AND MEDITATION

The work reported above indicates that during running and meditation there occurs a variety of endocrine, peripheral and subjective change. The absence of investigation into the higher level HPA hormones, 6-EP and CRH, during meditation stands out. A study by Harte (unpublished data) was designed, in part, to fill this gap and also to investigate trained runners and meditators, matched for age, personality and sex, in one experiment. A slight but insignificant change in plasma cortisol was found after subjects ran for an hour, and immunoreactive 6-EP (6-EP-IR) rose significantly during this condition. No change in cortisol or 6-EP-IR was evident after meditation. However, CRH-IR rose significantly after both the run and meditation. Further, 6-EP-IR and CRH-IR were significantly correlated with a change in positive affect in both cases. The rise in 6-EP-IR, it seems, was related to the hypermetabolic state associated with running, but this is discounted for CRH-IR, which increased after subjects engaged in both hypermetabolic and hypometabolic activities. To summarise, this study controlled the possibility of mediation by peripheral parameters, and CRH-IR was still observed. Why CRH-IR was not also involved in 6-EP and cortisol release during meditation is discussed in the next section.

V. CONCLUDING REMARKS

To summarise the findings reviewed here, psychoneuroendocrine concomitants of running include the release of catecholamines, cortisol, 6-EP-IR and CRH-IR, as well as positive affective change. By studying meditation, the hypermetabolic effects of physical exertion can be eliminated, and findings here revealed a link between positive affective change and urinary noradrenaline release and cortisol decrease. Although plasma 6-EP-IR and cortisol failed to show a change in a later study of meditation, CRH-IR not only increased, but correlated with positive affect. Attention was shown to mediate these responses in running and meditation. These findings generally illustrate the interplay between psychological and endocrine variables in two emotion-eliciting activities, adding credence to the heuristic model of emotion presented earlier.

The theoretical implications of these findings can be discussed in terms the biochemical processes involved in the HPA, and also in terms of emotion as a psychoneuroendocrinological phenomenon. To address the biochemical level, two interesting cases were described whereas CRH and catecholamine but not 6-EP activity, was found during a quiescent, anti-stressful state. Predictably, during running, the HPA axis is stimulated, and this is reflected in the release of catecholamines, cortisol, 6-EP and CRH As it is generally thought that CRH is the main secretagogue of 6-EP, there appeared to be some mediating factor preventing 6-EP release during meditation. A similar effect may explain the release of noradrenaline and not adrenaline during meditation. One piece of research implicates the necessity of arginine vasopressin (AVP) in the CRH-6-EP relationship,[44] and it is possible that during meditation AVP was not released. Future research should be directed in this area.

The psychological and neuroendocrine changes found during the two cases discussed here were shown to obey the contraints of the heuristic model of emotion. The point made here is that emotion is a general response which is basically a CNS reaction capable of l) self stimulation, 2) mediation by variables such as environment and attention, and 3) both mediation by and effects upon peripheral physiological parameters. When these effects are considered as a response to stress, general adaptive neuroendocrine patterns are implied. Remembering, however, that the running and meditation induced emotional effects described here are not borne of pathological conditions, to discuss the practical applications of these findings, there must be a link made between these effects and clinical stress. Consider, then, the model presented in Figure 3. According to this model, stress conditions are represented at the negative end of an emotional continuum, and psychoneuroendocrine responses aim to bring the organism toward homeostasis. Running and meditation are activities in which people

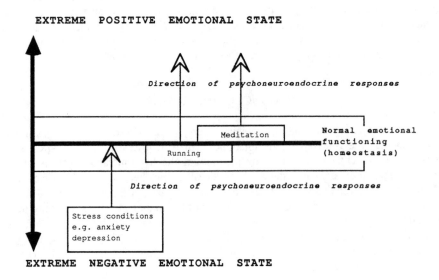

EXTREME POSITIVE EMOTIONAL STATE

Direction of psychoneuroendocrine responses

Meditation

Running

Normal emotional functioning (homeostasis)

Direction of psychoneuroendocrine responses

Stress conditions e.g. anxiety depression

EXTREME NEGATIVE EMOTIONAL STATE

Figure 3 An adaptive process. A metaphoric illustration of the relationship between stres-
induced and running/meditation-induced psychoneuroendocrine responses.

who are functioning within a normal homeostatic range engage, by choice. The
psychoneuroendocrine changes associated with these activities aim to bring the organism into
a heightened emotional state.

The psychological benefits of sports and leisure actitivies have been discussed for
many years, but empirical research, such as that reviewed here, is only beginning to validate
these effects. The practical applications of this type of research lie in understanding stress
responses in normal and clinical cases. By encouraging people to regularly engage in certain
activities, with the backing of established psychoneuroendocrine research, the increasing
incidences of pathological stress and associated depressive conditions may be attenuated.

VI. REFERENCES

1.   Selye, H., The evaluation of the stress concept-stress and cardiovascular disease, in
      Society, Stress and Disease, Levi, H., Ed., Oxford University Press, London, 1971.

2.   Lazarus, R.S., The concepts of stress and disease, in *Society, Stress and Disease*, Levi, L., Ed., Oxford University Press, London, 1971.

3.   Cannon, W.B., *Bodily Changes in Pain, Hunger, Fear and Rage*, Appelton-Century-Crofts, New York, 1915.

4.   James, W.T., The physical basis of the emotions, *Psychol.Rev.*, 1, 516, 1894.

5.   Calkins, M.W., *The Persistent Problems of Philosophy*, Macmillan, New York, 1925.

6.   Meyer, M., The nervousness correlates of pleasantness and unpleasantness, *Psychol.Rev.*, 15, 201, 1908.

7.   Frankenhaeuser, M., Experimental approaches to the study of catecholamines and emotion, in *Emotions: Their Parameters and Measurement*, Levi, L., Ed., Raven, New York, 1975.

8.   Selye, H., A syndrome produced by diverse nocuous agents, *Nature(Lond.)*, 138(32), 32, 1936.

9.   Smith, G.P., Adrenal hormones and emotional behaviour, in *Progress in Physiological Psychology*, Stellar, E. and Sprague, J.M., Eds., Academic Press, New York, 1973. 299.

10.   Brown, W.A. and Heninger, G., Cortisol, growth hormone, free fatty acids and experimentally induced affective arousal, *Am.J.Psychiatr.*, 132, 1172, 1975.

11.   Cannon, W.B., The mechanism of emotional disturbance of bodily function, *New Eng.J.Med.*, 198, 877, 1928.

12.   Greenspan, F.S. and Forsham, P.H., *Basic and Clinical Endocrinology*, Lange Medical Publications, Los Altos,Ca., 1983.

13.   Cohen, S.I. and Ross, R.N., *Handbook of Clinical Psychobiology and Pathology. Vol. 1*, Hemisphere, Washington, 1983.

14.   Gold, P.E. and McGaugh, J.L., Hormones and memory, in *Neuropeptide Influences on the Brain and Behavior*, Miller, L.H., Sandman, G.A. and Kasten, A.J., Eds., Raven Press, New York, 1977.

15.   Miller, L.H., Kastin, A.J., Sandman, C.A., Fink, M. and van Veen, W.J., Polypeptide influences on attention, memory and anxiety in man, *Pharmacol.Biochem.Behav.*, 2, 663, 1974.

16.   Taylor, A.L. and Fishman, L.M., Corticotropin-releasing hormone, *New Eng.J.Med.*, 319(4), 213, 1988.

17.   Staats, A. and Eifert, G.H., The paradigmatic behaviorism theory of emotions: basis for unification, *Clin.Psych.Rev.*, 10, 539, 1990.

18.   Barhke, M.S. and Morgan, W.P., Anxiety reduction following exercise and meditation, in *Psychology of Running*, Sacks, M.H. and Sachs, M.L., Eds., Human Kinetics Inc., Champaign, 1981.

19.   Greist, J.H., Klein, M.H., Eishens, R.R., Faris, J., Gurman, A.S. and Morgan, W.P., Running through your mind, in *Psychology of running*, Sacks, M.H. and Sachs, M.L., Eds., Human Kinetics Inc., Champaign, 1981.

20.   Kostrabula, T., *The Joy of Running*, J.B. Lippincott & Co., New York, 1976.

21.   Morgan, W.P., Psychophysiology of self awareness during vigorous physical activity, *Res.Q.Exerc.Sport*, 52(3), 385, 1981.

22.   Morgan, W.P., Psychological effects of exercise, *Behav.Med.Update*, 4(1), 25, 1982.

23.   Morgan, W.P., Affective beneficience of vigorous physical activity, *Med.Sci.Sports Exerc.*, 17(1), 94, 1985.

24.   Blaney, P.H., Affect and memory: a review, *Psychol.Bull.*, 99(2), 229, 1986.

25.   Joseph, P. and Robbins, J.M., Worker or runner? The impact of commitment to running and work on self-identification, in *Psychology of Running*, Sacks, M.H. and Sachs, M.L., Eds., Human Kinetics Inc. Champaign,III, 1981. 131.

26.   Sachs, M.L., Running addiction, in *Psychology of Running*, Sacks, M.H. and Sachs, M.L., Eds., Human Kinetics Inc., Champaign, 1981. 116.

27.   Sacks, M.H., Running addiction: a clinical report, in *Psychology of Running*, Sacks, M.H. and Sachs, M.L., Eds., Human Kinetics Inc., Champaign, 1981.

28.   Harte, J.L., Sports phenomenology: an application for a multi-levelled model of emotion, in *Proceedings of the 7th World Congress in Sports Psychology*, Giam, C.K., Chook, K.K. and Teh, K.C., Eds., I.S.S.P., Singapore, 1989. 192.

29.   Powers, S.K., Howley, E.T. and Cox, R., A differential catecholamine response during prolonged exercise and passive heating, *Med.Sci.Sports Exerc.*, 14(6), 435, 1982.

30.   Ransford, C.P., A role for amines in the anti-depressant effect of exercise: a review, *Med.Sci.Sports Exerc.*, 14(1), 1, 1982.

31.   Harte, J.L., Cortisol as an indicator of physical and mental stress in vigorous exercise. Paper presented at the annual conference of the Australasian Society for Human Biology,Canberra, 1989.

32.   Carr, D.B., Bullen, B.A., Skrinar, G.S., Arnold, M.A., Rosenblatt, M., Beitins, I.Z., Martin, J.B. and McArthur, J.W., Physical conditioning facilitates the exercise-induced secretion of β-lipoprotein in women, *New Eng.J.Med.*, 305, 560, 1981.

33.   Colt, E.W.D., Wardlaw, S.L. and Frank, A.G., The effect of running on plasma β-endorphin, *Life Sci.*, 28, 1637, 1981.

34.   Fraoli, F., Moretti, C., Paolucci, D., Alicicco, E., Crescenzi, F. and Fortunio, G., Physical exercise stimulates marked concomitant release of β- endorphin and adrenocorticotropic hormone (ACTH) in peripheral blood in man, *Experientia*, 36, 987, 1980.

35.   Gambert, S.R., Hagen, T.C., Garthwaite, T.L., Duthie, E.H. and McCarthy, D.J., Exercise and the endogenous opioids, *New Eng.J.Med.*, 305(26), 1590, 1981.

36.   Haier, R.J., Quaid, K. and Mills, J.S.C., Naloxone alters pain perception after jogging, *Psychiatr.Res.*, 5, 231, 1981.

37.   Janal, M.N., Colt, E.W., Clark, W.C. and Glusman, M., Pain sensitivity, mood and plasma endocrine levels in man following long distance running: effects of naloxone, *Pain*, 19(1), 13, 1984.

38.   Surbey, G.D., Andrew, G.M., Cervenko, F.W. and Hamilton, P.P., Effects of naloxone on exercise performance, *J.Appl.Physiol.*, 57(3), 674, 1984.

39.   Markoff, R.A., Ryan, P. and Young, T., Endorphins and mood changes in long-distance running, *Med.Sci.Sports Exerc.*, 14(1), 11, 1982.

40.   Jevning, R., Wilson, A., Vanderlaan, E. and Levine, S., Plasma prolactin and cortisol during transcendental meditation, in *Scientific Research on the TM Program: Collected Papers. Volume 1*, OrmeJohnson, D.W. and Farrow, J.T., Eds., Meru Press Publication, Geneva, 1975. 145.

41.   Bujatti, M. and Riederer, P., Serotonin, noradrenaline and dopamine metabolites in the transcendental meditation technique, *J.Neural Transm.*, 39, 257, 1976.

42.   Udupa, K.N., Singh, R.H. and Settiwar, R.M., Studies on physiological, endocrine and metabolic response to the practice of yoga in young normal volunteers, *J.Res.Ind.Med.*, 6(3), 345, 1971.

43.   Udupa, K.N., Singh, R.H., Settiwar, R.M. and Singh, M.B., Physiological and biochemical changes following the practice of some yogic and non-yogic exercises, *J.Res.Ind.Med.*, 10(2), 91, 1975.

44.   Burns, G., Almeida, O.F.X., Passarelli, F. and Herz, A., A two-step mechanism by which corticotropin releasing hormone releases hypothalamic β-endorphin: the role of vasopressin and G-proteins, *Endocrinology*, 125(3), 1365, 1989.

II. Conditioning of Immunity

CONDITIONING OF IMMUNOPHARMACOLOGICAL EFFECTS IN AUTO-IMMUNE DISEASES

Wolfgang Klosterhalfen and Sibylle Klosterhalfen

Institute of Medical Psychology,
University of Dusseldorf, Federal Republic of Germany

I. ABSTRACT

Using classical conditioning with immunosuppressive drugs, the course of two experimentally induced autoimmune diseases, systemic lupus erythematosus in mice, and adjuvant arthritis in rats, has been modified. In these studies cyclophosphamide or cyclosporine A has served as the unconditioned stimulus. The corresponding experiments are reviewed and their clinical implications are briefly discussed.

II. INTRODUCTION

Most experiments on the conditioning of immunopharmacologic effects have employed the taste aversion paradigm. In such experiments, rats or mice are presented with a distinctively flavored drinking solution (typically a saccharin solution), the consumption of which is followed by an injection of an immunomodulating drug (usually cyclophosphamide). The flavored solution is regarded as the conditioned stimulus (CS), and the immunomodulating drug the unconditioned stimulus (US). Reexposing animals to the CS usually results in conditioned taste aversion and in a conditioned attenuation of the immune response to some antigenic stimulation.[1-4]

Today, immunopharmacological conditioning effects are interesting for two major reasons: they provide us with a model to study neuroimmunologic interactions and they may be of clinical importance. We will focus on the latter aspect here and briefly review animal experiments in which the effects of conditioning on the course of autoimmune diseases were studied.

III. EFFECTS OF CONDITIONING ON LUPUS IN MICE

Ader and Cohen[5] were the first to test whether the course of a disease could be altered by an immunopharmacologic conditioning procedure (see Table 1). They chose systemic lupus erythematosus, an autoimmune disease that is spontaneously developed by female New Zealand hybrid mice (NZB x NZW). These animals show proteinuria and typically die within a few months after birth. Cyclophosphamide (Cy) and other immunosuppressive drugs delay the progression of disease. In the experiment to be discussed here, Group C50 received a total

Table 1 Reports on conditioning of immunopharmacological effects in experimental autoimmune disease.

Authors	Year	Exp.	CS	US	mg	subj.	model	CTA	results		p<
Ader, Cohen	1982	1	sac	Cy	30	mice	SLE	no	proteinuria days of life	→ ↑	.05 .05
Ader	1985	2	sac	Cy	30	mice	SLE	?	days of life	↑	?
Klosterhalfen, Klosterhalfen	1983	1	sac/van	Cy	100	rats	AA	yes	paw swelling	→	.01
		2	sac/van	Cy	80	rats	AA	yes	paw swelling	→	.01
Klosterhalfen, Klosterhalfen	1985	1	sac/van	Cy	80	rats	AA	yes	paw swelling	→	.01
		2	sac/van	Cy	100	rats	AA	yes	paw swelling	→	.001
		3	sac/van	Cy	30	rats	AA	yes	paw swelling	↑	.05
Klosterhalfen, Klosterhalfen	1990	1	Clm Vin	CyS	20	rats	AA	no	paw swelling	→	.01
		2	Clm Vin	CyS	20	rats	AA	no	paw swelling	→	.05

Note. CS = conditioned stimulus; Sac = saccharin; van = vanilla; Clm = cyclamate; Vin = vinegar; Cy = cyclophosphamide; CyS = cyclosporine A; SLE = systemic lupus erythemathosus; AA = adjuvant arthritis; CTA = conditioned taste aversion.

of 8 weekly intraperitoneal injections of Cy (US), half of these treatments being preceded by a presentation of a saccharin drinking solution (CS); Group NC50, the nonconditioned group, was subjected to the same pharmacologic treatment, however, exposure to saccharin and Cy was temporally separated. As expected on the basis of earlier "immunosuppressive" conditioning effects, in conditioned animals the rate of development of proteinuria and mortality were significantly retarded compared to nonconditioned animals. As the authors have pointed out, these data do not provide evidence of conditioned immunosuppression. "Nonetheless, the results are consistent with previous data[6] indicating that the pairing of saccharin and cyclophosphamide enables saccharin, acting as a CS, to suppress immunologic reactivity".[2]

The results of this important and frequently cited study were confirmed in a subsequent experiment.[1] In this study, the critical comparison is between Groups C33 and NC33. These groups were treated like Groups C5O and NC5O in the earlier report but with Cy injections every three weeks (on average) over a period of 12 weeks. In a second phase, saccharin alone was provided weekly until each animal's death. CS-presentations resulted again in a delay of mortality (level of significance not reported).

IV. EFFECTS OF CONDITIONING ON ARTHRITIS IN RATS

In a series of experiments (see Table 1) we studied the effects of conditioning on adjuvant arthritis (AA) in rats. With respect to histology, clinical characteristics, immunology, and pharmacology, AA has much in common with human rheumatoid arthritis.[7-9] This experimental disease can easily and reliably be induced by injecting complete Freund's adjuvant (heat-killed human mycobacterium tuberculosis suspended in light mineral oil) under light ether narcosis into a rat's hind paw. Paw swelling is the most prominent clinical symptom of AA. Depending on the amount of the adjuvant, the quality of the adjuvant, and the rat strain, not only the injected but - from about Day 12 after induction on - also the uninjected hind paw (and even the fore paws) may develop arthritic symptoms. To determine the degree of hind paw swelling, we used a scale of nine standards of acrylic-casted alginate impressions from arthritic hind paws (inter-rater correlations, r=0.85 - 0.95).[10]

In our first experiment,[11] we used a one-trial conditioning procedure with a high dose of Cy (i.p., 100 mg/kg) as the procedural US and a saccharin/vanilla drinking solution as the CS. CS-US pairing took place on Day -10 before the induction of AA (Group C); in nonconditioned controls the "CS" was presented on Day -12, the US two days later (Group NC). Groups C and NC received three unreinforced CS presentations on Days 0, 2, and 4; for an additional conditioned group, these CS presentations were on Days 2, 4, and 6 (Group C2). Ratings for the injected paws did not differ systematicaly between groups on Days 12 - 20. In contrast, no swelling occurred in the uninjected paws in Group C, whereas in the other two groups approximately half of the animals developed mild secondary lesions on Days 12-20.

In a second experiment, we used a lower dose of Cy (80 mg/kg) and obtained virtually the same results. The aim of the following experiments[12] was to inquire about the generality of conditioned immunopharmacologic effects in AA.

First we sought to demonstrate conditioning effects not only in the uninjected (op. cit.) but also in the injected hind paw. Therefore, the amount of adjuvant was reduced (as kindly suggested by R. Ader (pers. comm., 1983) from .1 to .05 ml. With this procedure, conditioned animals had less intense swellings of the injected hind paws, whereas the small swellings of the noninjected hind paws did not differ between Groups C and NC.

In a further experiment we assessed whether conditioning effects could be increased by a prolongation of the Cy-adjuvant interval to 5 wk (to decrease pharmacologic Cy effects on AA in both, conditioned and nonconditioned animals). Again, ratings for the injected paws were lower in Group C. Groups did not differ significantly with respect to the uninjected hind paws; only four rats in Group C and three rats in Group NC showed minor swellings.

The third experiment in this series tested whether the immunostimulating effects of a low dose of Cy[13] can be conditioned in AA. We therefore reduced the amount of Cy to 30 mg/kg. The swelling scores for the injected hind paws were higher in Group C than in Group NC on Days 12 to 20. In both groups, most of the animals developed small swellings at the uninjected hind paws; a rank test yielded no significant result.

In two recent experiments[14] we employed a differential conditioning design and used the immunosuppressive drug cyclosporine A (CyS; kindly provided by J. Borel, Sandoz, Basel, Switzerland) rather than Cy. One type of flavor (CS+) was seven times paired with CyS injections and another type of flavor (CS-) was never paired with the US. Following the acquisition period, half of the animals received unreinforced CS+ presentations, the other half CS- presentations. We found that in both, the injected and the noninjected hind paws, swelling was lower in rats tested with the CS + than in rats with the same history but tested with the CS-.

In a second experiment we changed the timing of the conditioning procedure in relation to the induction of AA and demonstrated "preventive" rather than "therapeutic" CS effects in the injected paws (the experiment was terminated before secondary swellings could develop).

In both experiments, animals showed a stable intake of the CS+ solution, that is, no indication of conditioned taste aversion. It should be noted, however, that CyS induced taste aversion has been observed by Neveu *et al*[15] and Grochowicz *etal*.[16]

V. DISCUSSION

Results from nine experiments demonstrate that the clinical course of systemic lupus erythematosus in mice and adjuvant arthritis in rats can be modified by conditioned stimuli that signal administration of an immunopharmacologic drug. These results confirm earlier reports on conditioned modulation of immunologic parameters[2] and extend them to two experimentally induced autoimmune diseases. These experiments show considerable methodological differences: as conditioned stimuli not only saccharin or a saccharin-vanilla combination were used but also vinegar and another artificial sweetener, cyclamate; in addition to cyclophosphamide, cyclosporine A constituted the US; different conditioning procedures, including a differential conditioning design, were employed; the temporal interval between acquisition and extinction as well as reinforcement rates varied. Despite these differences, results are remarkably consistent, both within and across the two autoimmune diseases that have been investigated.

It also seems important to point out that other immune related diseases have received much less attention so far. Obviously, (more) research is needed with respect to potential conditioning effects in experimentally induced allergies, cancer,[17] and infections. Patients with cancer or arthritis receive their medication repeatedly and typically in situations that contain sensory stimuli which reliably predict the administration of the pharmacologic US. It is therefore likely that the therapeutic as well as the adverse treatment effects seen in these patients include to a substantial degree conditioned drug effects. Clinically relevant conditioning effects in disease models are a good starting point to look for psycho-neuro-immuno-pathologic relationships. A better understanding of the psychologic and biologic mechanisms involved in conditioned immunopharmacologic effects may finally lead to improvements in the treatment of patients with immune related diseases.

VI. REFERENCES

1. Ader, R., Conditioned immunopharmacological effects in animals: Implications for a conditioning model of pharmacotherapy, in *Placebo: Theory, Research and Mechanisms*, White, L., Tursky, B. and Schwartz, G.E., Eds., Guilford, New York, 1985, 306.

2. Ader, R. and Cohen, N., The influence of conditioning on immune responses, in *Psychoneuroimmunology II*, Ader, R. and Cohen, N., Eds., Academic Press, Orlando, 1991.

3. Cresson, O., *Conditioning and the immune system: A guide to the data. Western Michigan University, Kalamazoo.*, 1990, unpublished.

4. Klosterhalfen, S. and Klosterhalfen, W., The conditioning of immunophannacologic effects: critical remarks and perspectives, in *Immuno-Neuro-Endocrine Network: Recent Research*, Jankovic, B.D., Ed., Gordon & Breach, New York, 1991, In press.

5. Ader, R. and Cohen, N., Behaviourally conditioned immunosuppression and murine systemic lupus erythematosus, *Science*, 215, 1534, 1982.

6. Ader, R. and Cohen, N., Behaviorally conditioned immunosuppression, *Psychosom.Med.*, 37, 333, 1975.

7. Pearson, C.M., Immunomodulation by behavioural conditioning, in *Arthritis and allied conditions*, McCarty, D.J., Ed., Lea & Febiger, Philadelphia, 1979.

8. Taurog, D., Argentieri, D.C. and McReynolds, R.A., Adjuvant arthritis, *Methods Enzymol.*, 162, 339, 1988.

9. Klosterhalfen, W. and Klosterhalfen, S., Stress effects in experimental models of arthritis, in *Immuno-Neuro-Endocrine Network:Recent Research*, Jankovic, B.D., Ed., Gordon & Breach, New York, 1991, in press.

10. Klosterhalfen, W., *Experimenteller Stress und Adjuvans-Arthritis: Ein Beitrag zur Psychoimmunologie (Experimental stress and adjuvant arthritis: A contribution to psychoimmunology)*, Athenaum, Frankfurt, 1987.

11. Klosterhalfen, W. and Klosterhalfen, S., Pavlovian conditioning of immunosuppression modified adjuvant arthritis in rats, *Behav.Neurosci.*, 97, 663, 1983.

12.   Klosterhalfen, S. and Klosterhalfen, W., Conditioned immunopharmacologic effects and adjuvant arthritis: Further results, in *Proceedings of the First International Workshop on Neuroimmunomodulation*, Spector, N.H., Ed., IWGN, Bethesda,MD, 1985, 183.

13.   Kayashima, K., Koga, T. and Onoue, K., Role of T lymphocytes in adjuvant arthritis. II. Different subpopulations of T lymphocytes functioning in the development of the disease, *J.Immunol.*, 120, 1127, 1978.

14.   Klosterhalfen, S. and Klosterhalfen, W., Conditioned cyclosporine effects but not conditioned taste averesion in immunized rats, *Behav.Neurosci.*, 104, 716, 1990.

15.   Neveu, P.J., Crestani, F. and Le Moal, M., Conditioned immunosuppression: A new methodological approach, *Ann.N.Y.Acad.Sci.*, 496, 595, 1987.

16.   Grochowicz, P., Schedlowski, M., Husband, A.J., King, M.G., Hibberd, A.D. and Bowen, K.M., Behavioral conditioning prolongs heart allograft survival in rats, *Brain Behav.Immun.*, 1991.(In Press)

17.   Ghanta, V., Hiramoto, R.N., Solvason, B. and Spector, N.H., Influence of conditioned natural immunity on tumor growth, *Ann.N.Y.Acad.Sci.*, 496, 637, 1987.

HEART ALLOGRAFT SURVIVAL PROLONGED BY
BEHAVIOURAL CONDITIONING

M. Schedlowski[a], P. Grochowicz[b], A.J. Husband[c], M.G. King[d],
K.M. Bowen[e] & A.D. Hibberd[b]

[a]Department of Medical Psychology, Medical School Hannover, FRG; [b]Department of
Transplantation Medicine, The Royal Newcastle Hospital, Newcastle; [c]Faculty of Medicine
and [d]Department of Psychology, The University of Newcastle, Newcast]e; [e]Department of
Endocrinology, The Royal Newcastle Hospital, Newcastle, Australia.

I. ABSTRACT

The purpose of this study was to investigate whether behavioral conditioned
immunosupression is able to prolong graft rejection of a vascularized organ allograft in the
rat. Using the paradigm of heterotopic heart transplantation male DA rats received a Lewis
rat cardiac allograft. The recipients were randomly allocated to one of 5 groups. The
conditioning groups received 2 conditioned trials on day 10 and on day 6 prior to
transplantation with either water or saccharin as the conditioned stimulus (CS) and an
injection of Cyclosporin A (CsA) or phosphate buffered saline as the unconditioned stimulus
(UCS). One day prior to transplantation the rats were reexposed to the CS alone. The next
day the heart transplantation was performed. On day 3 following surgery the rats were re-
exposed a second time to the CS. After day 3 the water deprivation ceased and cardiac
activity was assessed daily by abdominal palpation and ECG recording. The experimental
conditioning group which received saccharin as the CS and CsA as the UCS developed a taste
aversion against the saccharin and showed a significant prolongation of heart graft survival
compared to the conditioned and non-conditioned control groups.

II. INTRODUCTION

Emperical evidence now exists which shows that the immune system is connected to
the central nervous system (CNS) directly and/or indirectly via the neuroendocrine system.[1-3]
One approach to the study of these bidirectional interactions is behavioural conditioning of
immunopharmacological effects using a conditioned taste aversion regimen. In this variation
of the paradigm of classical conditioning, thirsty animals drink a novel tasting solution
(conditioning stimulus/CS) after which they receive an intraperitoneal injection of an
immunosuppressive drug (unconditioned stimulus/UCS). On re-exposure to the CS alone,
animals exhibit a conditioned taste aversion against the CS and the CS re-enlists
immunosuppressive properties of the UCS.

Since the initial study of Ader & Cohen[4] who reported reduced serum antibody titers
to sheep red blood cells (RBC) in rats after taste aversion conditioning with

cyclophosphamide, a number of studies have demonstrated conditioned modulation of immune functions. For example, reduced mixed lymphocyte culture reactivity,[5] a suppression of graft-vs-host response,[6] reduced mitogen-induced lymphoproliferation.[7] That behavioural conditioning can also be a useful regimen to enhance the immune functions is shown from studies which have reported an increase in the activity of natural killer cells[8] or increased helper:suppressor T cell subset ratio after taste aversion conditioning with levamisole.[9]

Although the clinical implications of behavioural immunomodulation are still a matter of issue, a few studies have reported clinical impact of conditioned immunosuppression. Ader & Cohen[10] found a reduced rate of mortality from systemic lupus erythematosus, an auto-immune disease, when CY was paired with the CS without inducing taste aversion. A reduction of adjuvant-induced arthritis in rats by using taste aversion with CY was reported by Klosterhalfen & Klosterhalfen[11] and Ghanta *et al*[12] demonstrated that camphor odour as the CS paired with poly I:C as the UCS leads to a decreased growth of transplanted tumour and increased survival in mice.

Organ transplantation, similar to autoimmune diseases is one of the most important clinical situations in which the suppression of the immune system is required. The purpose of this study was to determine whether behavioral conditioned immunosupression is able to prolong graft rejection of a vascularized organ allograft.

III. MATERIALS AND METHODS

We used the paradigm of heterotopic heart transplantation[13] which is a standardized model used in various immunological investigations. Briefly, the donor heart is anastomosed in the recipient's abdomen by end to side anastomosis of the donors aorta to the recipient's aorta and the donor pulmonary vein to the inferior vena cava of the recipient. In this way the blood is allowed to flow from the recipients aorta in the coronary arteries of the transplanted heart, thus nourishing the heart. Blood is then drained via the coronary veins into the right atrium, from here to the right ventricle and then pumped out from the right ventricle into the pulmonary artery to the vena cava of the recipient, whereby the blood is completely bypassing the left ventricle. Such a heart beats normally and is nourished normally. The blood flow through the transplanted heart is approximately 5% of the total blood volume per minute.[14] The function and the rejection time of the transplanted heart can be precisely monitored by palpation and ECG recording. A progressive slowing of heart rate and appearance of an idio-ventricular rhythm, and finally cardiac arrest, follows the rejection.

We used Cyclosporin A (CsA) as the UCS in this study since it has potent immunosuppressive properties and is in current clinical use to prevent graft rejection.[15] CsA acts relatively selectively on T lymphocytes in an early stage of T-cell activation mainly by blocking the release of interleukin-2 (IL-2) and other lymphokines from T-helper cells.[16]

Adult male DA rats weighing 230-250 g received adult Lewis rat cardiac allograft. The recipients were conditioned according to the protocol shown in Figure 1.

The conditioned groups received 2 conditioned trials on day 10 and on day 6 prior to transplantation. Either water or .2% of saccharin (sacc) diluted in tap water served as the

CS. The UCS was an intraperitoneal injection of CsA (20mg/kg) dissolved in 1ml phosphate buffered saline (PBS) or 1ml of pure PBS as control. One day prior to transplantation the rats were re-exposed to the CS alone. The next day the heart transplantation was performed. On day 3 after the operation rats were re-exposed a second time to the CS. After day 3 the water deprivation ceased and cardiac activity was assessed daily by palpation which was confirmed by electrocardiogram recording.

The graft recipients were randomly allocated to one of 5 groups. Group A, the experimental group, received sacc as the CS and CsA as the UCS. Group B, control for the residual effects of CsA was given water as the CS and CsA as the UCS. Group C served as a control for the non-specific conditioned response to injection and handling and received sacc and PBS as a CS/UCS combination. Group D, control for the non-specific effects of the CS, received water as the CS and PBS as a UCS. Group E served as a non treated / non-conditioned control group.

We hypothesized on the basis of the previous results of behavioral conditioned immunosuppression that a taste aversion to sacc and a prolongation of heart graft survival in the experimental Group A compared to the control groups would occur.

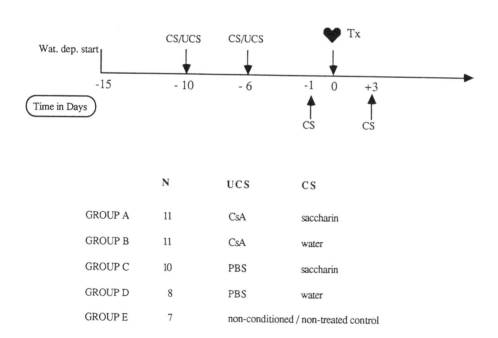

Figure 1. Conditioning protocol and treatment groups summary.

IV. RESULTS

Figure 2 shows the mean fluid consumption on the conditioning trials 10 and 6 days prior to transplantation and at the re-exposure to sacc alone 1 day prior to and 3 days after transplantation for the conditioned groups. The behavioural responses display a taste aversion for group A against the CS (sacc) compared to the control groups starting from the first re-exposure to the sacc on day -6. ANOVA revealed a significant group effect [$F(3,36)$ = 38.06; $p < .00l$], a significant time [$F(3,108)$ = 3.56; $p < .02$] and a significant (group x time) interaction effect [$F(3,108)$ = 6.02; $p < .00l$]. The groups which were exposed to the sacc on day -10 (group A and group C) drank significantly less fluid compared to the water groups (B and C) [$t(38)$ = -3.06; $p < .0l$] demonstrating a characteristic neophobic response to the sacc solution.

The Cumulative Rejection Rate of heart grafts is shown in Figure 3. Wilcoxon rank-sum analysis (one-tailed) of the heart graft survival time (defined as the last day of palpable cardiac activity) revealed a significant difference between Group A and each of the control groups (A vs B $p < .02$ / A vs C $p < .03$ / A vs D .$p < .02$ / A vs E $p < .0l$). Indeed, in one animal in Group A the graft was functioning perfectly even after day 100 post transplantation. This animal apparently developed a complete immunological tolerance against the major histocompatibility complex (MHC) incompatible heart graft. But even excluding this animal from the statistical analysis, the differences between group A and the control groups remain significant ($p < .05$). Although the influence of regulated water acces on adrenal cortex

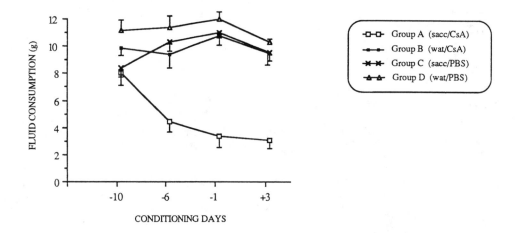

Figure 2. Mean consumption of CS (0.2% saccharin or tap water) on the conditioning trials 10 and 6 days prior to the transplantation and at re-exposure to the CS alone 1 day prior to and 3 days after transplantation for the conditioned groups.

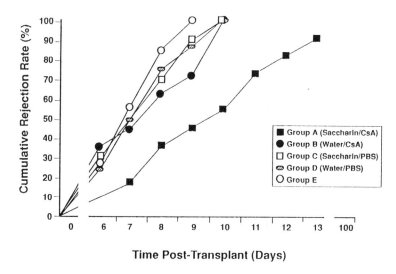

Figure 3. Cumulative Rejection Rate of Lewis donor hearts by DA recipients, wher heart graft survival defined as the last day of palpable cardiac activity.

activity in the rat is minimal some authors reported effects of water restriction on circadian rhythms of this hormone.[17] Nonetheless an untreated/nonconditioned control group (Group E) received heart allografts. The rejection time in this group displayed the same pattem as the other control groups.

V. DISCUSSION

This study was conducted to determine whether the rejection of a heart allograft in a MHC incompatible model could be prolonged by behaviourally conditioned immunosuppression. Using the heterotopic heart transplantation model and CsA as an UCS the results show a taste aversion against the CS in the experimental conditioning group A and a significant prolongation of heart graft survival in this group compared to the conditioned control groups.

The underlying mechanismen for these effects remains unclear however there are several possibilities. In concensus with the studies reporting behaviourally conditioned immunosuppression the prolongation of heart graft survival could be attributed to the conditioning process, more specifically to the ability of the CS to re-enlist the immunosuppressive propertics of CsA. Eikelboom & Stewart[18] have provided a functional model of conditioned drug effects. These authors have stressed that when a drug, used as an UCS, is stimulating the afferent arm of the CNS the CR will mimic the primary response of the drug. If, however, the drug is acting on the efferent arm of the CNS the CR will counteract the drug effects. Our results fit into this functional model of a CNS-mediated conditioned drug effects and support the assumption of an immune system-CNS interaction.

Although the results of this *in vivo* study provide no direct evidence for neuro-immune interactions *per se*, the specific immunosuppressive effects of CsA supports the proposition that lymphokines seems to be an important factor for the bidirectional communication between the immune system and the CNS.

The phenomen of organ allograft rejection is a highly complex process where the interaction between antigen presenting cells, CD4 (helper/inducer) cells and CD8 (cytotoxic) cells are mainly responsible for rejection of MHC incompatible grafts.[19] There is now a general agreement that CsA suppresses the production and release of many lymphokines, especially IL-2 and interferon-γ from CD4 T-cells and inhibits the activation of CD8 T-cells at an early stage and is able to protect the allograft.[20,21] Lymphokines are known to be active in the CNS and on various neuroendocrine dssues.[22,23] The administradon of CsA causes a decrease of lymphokine levels which might act on the CNS directly and/or through an indirect way via mediators produced by the neuroendocrine system. The same feedback loop is quite likely to be activated after the reexposure to the CS alone.[24,25] However further investigations which include the analyses of lymphokine levels have to determine whether the CS leads to an inhibition of lymphokine release similar to the observed effects of CsA.

Because of the reduced Cs intake in the experimental group A another explanation for the prolonged heart graft survival in this group might be that, that the taste aversion paradigm induces a stress response with enhanced adrenocortical activity which finally leads to immunosuppression.[26] However there is now compelling data that the conditioned modulation of immune functions can not simply be traced back to an enhanced release of adrenal cortex hormones, indicating that it is more likely that the CS is able to re-enlist the benificial effects of the drug.[27-30] Furthermore in this study there is no correlation ($r < .03$) between the CS consumption and the graft survival time in the experimental Group A.

With this first attempt to prolong the rejection time of heart allograft by using a behavioural conditioned immunosuppression regimen we received as a result a significant prolongation of graft survival time in our treatment group compared to the control groups. However the differences are small and at this stage one can only speculate about the clinical application of this method in human transplantation medicine. But of particular interest in this context can be a partial reinforcement strategy of drug administration which could be an effective procedure for reducing the amount of toxic drug effects while maximizing therapeutic efficacy.

VI. REFERENCES

1. Ader, R., *Psychoneuroimmunology*, Academic Press, New York, 1981.
2. Besedovsky, H.O. and del Rey, A., Immune-neuroendocrine network, *Progr.Immunol.*, 6, 578, 1986.
3. Blalock, J.E., A molecular basis for bidirectional communication between the immune and neuroendocrine systems, *Physiol.Rev.*, 69, 1, 1989.
4. Ader, R. and Cohen, N., Behaviorally conditioned immunosuppression, *Psychosom.Med.*, 37, 333, 1975.
5. Kusnecov, A.W., Sivyer, M., King, M.G., Husband, A.J., Cripps, A.W. and Clancy, R.L., Behaviorally conditioned suppression of the immune response by

antilymphocyte serum, *J.Immunol.*, 130, 2117, 1983.

6. Bovbjerg, D., Ader, R. and Cohen, N., Acquisition and extinction of conditioned suppression of a graft- vs-host response in the rat, *J.Immunol.*, 132, 111, 1984.

7. Neveu, R.J., Dantzer, R. and Le Moal, M., Behaviorally conditioned immunosuppression of mitogen-induced lymphoproliferation and antibody production in mice, *Neurosci.Lett.*, 65, 293, 1986.

8. Ghanta, V.K., Hiramoto, R.M., Solvason, H.B. and Spector, N.H., Neural and environmental influences on neoplasia and conditioning of NK activity, *J.Immunol.*, 135(Suppl.), 848s, 1985.

9. Husband, A.J., King, M.G. and Brown, R., Behaviourally conditioned modification of T cell subset ratios in rats, *Immunol.Lett.*, 14, 91, 1987.

10. Ader, R. and Cohen, N., Behaviourally conditioned immunosuppression and murine systemic lupus erythematosus, *Science*, 215, 1534, 1982.

11. Klosterhalfen, W. and Klosterhalfen, S., Pavlovian conditioning of immunosuppression modified adjuvant arthritis in rats, *Behav.Neurosci.*, 97, 663, 1983.

12. Ghanta, V.K., Hiramoto, R.M., Solvason, H.B. and Spector, N.H., Influence of conditioned natural immunity on tumor growth, *Ann.N.Y.Acad.Sci.*, 496, 637, 1987.

13. Ono, K. and Lindsey, E.S., Improved technique of heart transplantation in rats, *J.Thorac.Cardiovasc.Surg.*, 7, 225, 1969.

14. Silber, S.J., *Microsurgery*, Williams and Wilkins, Baltimore, 1979.

15. Green, C.J., Experimental Transplantation and Cyclosporine, *Transplantation*, 46(Suppl.), 3, 1988.

16. Thomson, A.W., *Cyclosporin*, Kluwer Academic Publishers, London, 1989.

17. Armario, A. and Jolin, T., Effects of water restriction on circadian rhythms of corticosterone, growth hormone and thyroid stimulating hormone in adult male rats, *Physiol.Behav.*, 38, 327, 1986.

18. Eikelboom, R. and Stewart, J., Conditioning of drug-induced physiological responses, *Psychol.Rev.*, 89, 507, 1982.

19. Tilney, N.L. and Kupiec-Weglinski, J.W., Advances in the understanding of rejection mechanisms, *Transplant.Proc.*, 21, 10, 1989.

20. Granelli-Piperno, A., Inaba, K. and Steinman, R.M., Stimulation of Lymphokine release from T lymphoblasts- requirement for mRNA synthesis and inhibiton by CsA, *J.exp.Med.*, 160, 1792, 1984.

21. Ryffel, B., Tammi, K., Grieder, A. and Hess, A.D., Effects of cyclosporine on human T cell activation, *Transplant.Proc.*, 17, 1268, 1985.

22. Pert, C.B., Ruff, M.R., Weber, R.J. and Herkenham, M., Neuropeptides and their receptors: A psychosomatic network, *J.Immunol.*, 135, 820s, 1985.

23. Brown, S.L., Smith, L.R. and Blalock, J.E., Interleukin 1 and interleukin 2 enhance proopiomelanocortin gene expression in pituitary cells, *J.Immunol.*, 139, 3181, 1987.

24. Hall, N.R., McGillis, J.P., Spangelo, B.L. and Goldstein, A.L., Evidence that thymosins and other biologic responsemodifiers can function as neuroactive immunotransmitters, *J.Immunol.*, 135, 806, 1985.

25. Neveu, P.J., Crestani, F. and Le Moal, M., Conditioned immunosuppression: A new methodological approach, *Ann.N.Y.Acad.Sci.*, 496, 595, 1987.

26. Kelley, K.W., Dantzer, R., Mormede, P., Salmon, H. and Aynaud, J.M., Conditioned taste aversion suppresses induction of delayed-type hypersensitivity immune reactions, *Physiol.Behav.*, 34, 189, 1985.

27.   Ader, R., Cohen, N. and Grota, L.J., Adrenal involvement in conditioned immunosuppression, *Int.J.Immunopharmacol.*, 1, 141, 1979.

28.   King, M.G., Husband, A.J. and Kusnecov, A.W., Behaviorally conditioned immunosuppression using antilymphoctye serum: Duration of effect and role of corticosteroids, *Med.Sci.Res.*, 15, 407, 1987.

29.   Klosterhalfen, S. and Klosterhalfen, W., Classically conditioned effects of cyclophosphamide on white blood cell counts in rats, *Ann.N.Y.Acad.Sci.*, 496, 569, 1987.

30.   Kusnecov, A.W., Husband, A.J. and King, M.G., The influence of dexamethasone on behaviorally conditioned immunomodulation and plasma corticosterone, *Brain Behav.Immun.*, 4, 50, 1990.

CONDITIONED ALLERGIC RHINITIS: A MODEL FOR CENTRAL NERVOUS SYSTEM AND IMMUNE SYSTEM INTERACTION IN IgE-MEDIATED ALLERGIC REACTIONS

M. Gauci, A.J. Husband, & M.G. King[a]

Faculty of Medicine and [a]Department of Psychology,
University of Newcastle. NSW. 2308. Australia.

I. ABSTRACT

This study has investigated the potential for allergic rhinitis (AR) to be induced as a conditioned response, assessed by clinical symptoms and tosyl-1-arginine methyl ester esterase (TE) activity. Twenty seven allergic subjects participated. On conditioning days, Group 1 subjects (n=9) were given a novel drink as a conditioned stimulus (CS) paired with allergen challenge as the unconditioned stimulus (UCS). On the test day, subjects received the novel drink paired with allergen-free PBS. Group 2 subjects (n=9) received novel drink paired with PBS on conditioning days and test day. Group 3 subjects (n=9) consumed tap water paired with allergen on conditioning days and tap water paired with PBS on test day. Analysis of TE activity showed that on test day enzyme activity differed among the groups (χ^2 = 6.321, d.f.= 2, $p < 0.05$)(Kruskal-Wallace). TE activity was greater in Group 3 compared with Group 2 ($p < 0.05$) but was not significantly different between Groups 1 and 2. These results suggested that a generalised conditioning effect had occurred in Group 3, that is, conditioning to aspects of the environment other than the novel drink CS. The large heterogeneity of variance contributed by Group 1 on test day ($\chi^2 = 31.42$, d.f.=2, $p < 0.05$) (Bartlett[1]) indicated that the novel drink had a bi-modal effect on the conditioning of AR. The results of this study implicate roles for conditioning, expectation, and the placebo effect in the management of allergic disorders.

II. INTRODUCTION

Evidence has accumulated since 1964 which supports the speculative hypothesis introduced by Solomon & Moos[2] that there is a bi-directional interaction between the immune system and the central nervous system (CNS). For example the work of Shavit et al,[3] Kraut & Greenberg[4] and Kusnecov et al,[5,6] showed that neuropeptides influenced immune reactivity while other studies demonstrated that immune reactivity affected neurological activity (e.g. Besedovsky et al,[7] Del Ray et al,[8] Harbour-McMenamin et al.[9]

An important contribution to this growing body of research is provided by studies in which behavioural conditioning has modified a variety of immunological parameters. For example, behaviourally conditioned immuno-augmentation has been demonstrated to occur in several effector arms of the immune system, including numbers of cytotoxic T cell precursors;[10] natural killer cell activity;[11] delayed type hypersensitivity;[12] and helper:suppressor T cell subset ratios.[13]

Similarly, behaviourally conditioned immuno-suppression has been documented for a number of humoral and cell-mediated immune responses.[14-17]

Most studies of behavioural conditioning of immunity have employed classical Pavlovian conditioning techniques[18] to train animals to elevate or suppress immune responses. These suggest that the animal learns to associate exposure to a conditioned stimulus (CS) (i.e. a sensory cue such as a novel-tasting drinking solution), with an unconditioned stimulus (UCS) (i.e. an immunomodulatory agents given to the animal immediately following the CS. The immunomodulatory effect is then re-enlisted on subsequent exposure to the CS alone.[19]

The potential for clinical benefits of behaviourally conditioned immunomodulation in human health are far-reaching. For example, behavioral conditioning may be used to counteract the anticipatory nausea associated with cancer chemotherapy.[20,21] Similarly, behavioural conditioning may have important implications for re-enlisting the therapeutic effects of drugs used by AIDS patients or immunosuppressive drugs used in tissue transplantation, whilst reducing detrimental side-effects associated with the drugs.[10,22]

A limited number of studies have also been reported in which behavioural conditioning of allergic reactions has been effected. In the earliest recorded case study, MacKenzie[23] noted that a patient allergic to roses experienced symptoms of allergy when presented with an artificial rose. Similarly, Dekker and Groen[24] reported that one subject who developed asthma attacks when viewing a goldfish in a bowl incurred allergic symptoms when shown a picture of the goldfish. In addition, two allergic individuals who were exposed to allergens when using a breathing apparatus exhibited allergic symptoms when using the breathing apparatus alone.[25] These single case studies suggested that the individuals had associated the offending allergen (UCS) with a specific visual cue (CS) with the result that allergic reactions could be re-enlisted upon subsequent exposure to the CS alone.

A more recent study showed that it was possible to condition suppression of delayed-type allergic responses (a measure of cell-mediated immunity) to the tuberculin allergen in healthy subjects. By using the colour of the vial containing either tuberculin or saline as a CS, it was possible to elicit a decreased response to the allergen when the vial colour associated with tuberculin on all previous trials was switched to that associated with saline on the final trial.[26]

In another study, Russell *et al*[27] showed that histamine was released into the plasma when guinea pigs were exposed to an odour (CS) alone after having been initially conditioned by an allergen challenge (UCS) paired with the odour.

Finally, MacQueen *et al*[28] showed that rat mast cell protease II, a mediator of allergic reactions, was released from mast cells when exposure to allergen (UCS) was paired with an audiovisual cue (CS) and that this response was re-enlisted upon exposure to the CS alone.

The above studies implicate a role for CNS involvement in initiating allergic responses via Pavlovian conditioning mechanisms. It was the aim of this study to further investigate the role of classical conditioning in allergic reactions. Allergic rhinitis (AR) was selected as the allergic disorder to be conditioned. AR is an IgE-mediated allergic disorder of the human nasal mucosa occurring perennially in response to dust or mold or seasonally in response to pollens and grasses (hay fever). Sufferers of this disease may experience a range of symptoms varying in severity including sneezing, rhinorrhea, nasal congestion, itchy eyes and throat.[29]

In this study allergen challenge (UCS) was paired with a novel-tasting, non-toxic, non-allergenic soft drink (CS) in a group of AR sufferers in an attempt to classically condition AR. Two indicators of AR: (1) clinical symptoms (as assessed by subjective symptom score [SSS]) and (2) release of mast cell mediators (as assessed by tosyl-1-arginine methyl ester esterase [TE] activity) were used. The latter indicator of AR was employed to ensure that the allergic symptoms observed were the result of mast cell degranulation because it is well documented that enzymes exhibiting TE activity are released from mast cells upon stimulation with allergen.[30,31]

The hypothesis was tested that after two training sessions where subjects were challenged with allergen immediately after consumption of the novel drink, expression of AR as indicated by TE activity and SSS would be re-enlisted upon subsequent exposure to the CS alone.

III. METHOD

A. SUBJECTS

Subjects of both sexes, 18 - 50 years of age were recruited and interviewed separately at the Royal Newcastle Hospital, Newcastle. Those who reacted positively on a standard skin prick test to at least one common allergen, and who were not excluded from the study according to an exclusion criteria list were eligible to complete the study. The first thirty subjects who fulfilled these criteria were selected for the study.

Subjects were randomly assigned into one of three treatment groups: (1) drink conditioned group (n=10); (2) control group (n=10); or (3) non-drink conditioned group (n=10).

B. MATERIALS AND PROCEDURES

An exclusion criteria list was completed for each subject which ascertained whether any recent medication was likely to affect immune responses. Skin prick tests were performed using standard allergen solutions (neat) to mold mix #4, grass mix #7 , and house dust mites *Dermatophagoides pteronyssinus* and *D. farinae* (all from Miles Inc., Elkhart, Indiana) as well as positive and negative control solutions (histamine [1mg/ml] and phosphate buffered saline [PBS] respectively). The diameters of the resulting indurations at the site of each allergen application were recorded. The novel flavoured drink was prepared daily by combining soda water, methyl anthranylate, benzaldehyde and methyl salicylate in the ratios 44 : 8 : 2 : 1 (400 ml per subject per session). Nasal allergen challenges were performed using the identical allergen solutions used in skin prick tests, sterile filtered and diluted 1:100 with PBS. Symptoms of AR were recorded on subjective symptom score sheets (SSS) before and after nasal challenge. Nasal washings (NW) were collected in sterile 50 ml containers in sterile normal saline (NS). TE activity from NW was measured using the technique described by Naclerio *et al*.[30]

The experimental room was arranged in an identical manner for all subjects in all sessions to minimise any environmental differences between sessions which may have interfered with conditioning. Protocols were performed on subjects individually to avoid any effects of interactions between subjects which may have influenced the outcome of the experiment. Procedures performed are outlined in Table 1. Identical procedures were carried out for each group unless otherwise indicated.

In the first session, (approximately 20 minutes duration), the exlusion criteria list was completed. Subjects for whom one or more exclusion criteria applied were excluded from further participation because results may have been confounded by recent medication or by an abnormal current immune status, for example, an upper respiratory tract infection. Eligible subjects were skin prick tested with common allergens according to standard procedures.

At the start of the second session (conditioning day 1 [CD1]), about 45 minutes duration, two 10ml NW were collected at 2 min intervals to determine baseline levels of TE. After collection, NWs were kept on ice to inhibit TE activity until the completion of the session when they were stored at -20°C until assayed.

Subjects then completed the pre-challenge SSS. After a 10 min time interval, subjects were offered 400 ml of the novel soft drink and requested to drink as much or as little as they chose. Immediately following drink consumption, subjects were informed that they were then going to be challenged with a dilute solution of the allergen to which they had tested most positive by skin prick test and that they may experience some hay fever-like symtoms. The subject was instructed to inhale through the nose as 50 μl of the appropriate allergen solution was delivered to each nostril with a disposable transfer pipette. Post-challenge NW's were collected 5 and 15 minutes following allergen administration and post-challenge SSS were completed at both of these times (Table 1).

It was necessary to collect both an early (5 minute) and a late (15 minute) post-challenge NW because subjects vary in their response to allergen challenge in terms of peak TE release and onset of clinical symptoms. A 5 minute and a 15 minute sample accomodated both early and late responders.[32]

Two days following CD1, the identical procedure was followed. This was conditioning day 2 (CD2), also 45 minutes duration (Table 1). The same protocol was performed on the test day (test day), (five days after CD2), except that allergen-free PBS was administered instead of allergen. Subjects were still informed, however, that they would receive a dose of allergen to which they might experience some hay fever-like symptoms. The above procedure was followed for Group 2 subjects (control group) except that they received the novel drink paired with allergen-free PBS on CD1, CD2, and test day. This group was defined as the control group because no peturbation of the immune response was effected i.e. these subjects received no allergen (UCS).

Table 1. Conditioning Protocols Performed on Subjects with Allergic Rhinitis

Group 1 (Drink-conditioned)

Ses-sion	Day	Procedure				
1		Skin test				
2	CD1	NW1	NW2/SSS	Drink/Allergen	NW3/SSS	NW4/SSS
3	CD2	NW1	NW2/SSS	Drink/Allergen	NW3/SSS	NW4/SSS
4	TD	NW1	NW2/SSS	Drink/PBS	NW3/SSS	NW4/SSS

Group 2 (Control)

Ses-sion	Day	Procedure				
1		Skin test				
2	CD1	NW1	NW2/SSS	Drink/PBS	NW3/SSS	NW4/SSS
3	CD2	NW1	NW2/SSS	Drink/PBS	NW3/SSS	NW4/SSS
4	TD	NW1	NW2/SSS	Drink/PBS	NW3/SSS	NW4/SSS

Group 3 (Non-Drink Conditioned)

Ses-sion	Day	Procedure				
1		Skin test				
2	CD1	NW1	NW2/SSS	Water/Allergen	NW3/SSS	NW4/SSS
3	CD2	NW1	NW2/SSS	Water/Allergen	NW3/SSS	NW4/SSS
4	TD	NW1	NW2/SSS	Water/PBS	NW3/SSS	NW4/SSS

CD = conditioning day; TD = test day; NW = nasal washing; SSS = subjective symptom score

Group 3 subjects (non-drink conditioned) were given tap water instead of the novel drink prior to challenge with allergen on CD1 and CD2. On test day, allergen-free PBS was administered after the water was drunk. As for Group 1 and 2 subjects, Group 3 subjects were asked to drink as much or as little water as they chose. Treatment of group 3 subjects enabled the effects of the UCS associated with conditioning stimuli other than the novel drink to be studied. For example, association of the UCS with particular objects or odours in the experimental room, features of the investigator, the expectation of an allergic response, or the suggestion of hay fever-like symptoms by the investigator may have influenced immune responses on test day. Conditioning to such uncontrolled cues would reflect a generalised conditioning phenomenon.

C. TE ACTIVITY

Briefly, TE in NW was reacted with a synthetic substrate (tosyl-1-arginine methyl ester) radiolabelled with tritium. The amount of tritiated methyl released into the organic phase of the reaction solution was measured in a beta scintillation counter and expressed as counts per minute (cpm). The mean triplicate assay value indicated TE activity present in each NW.[30]

Differences in TE activity before and after challenge with allergen or PBS were determined by subtracting the mean pre-challenge TE value (NW2) from the highest mean post-challenge TE value (i.e. either NW3 or NW4, 5 minutes or 15 minutes post-challenge respectively). NW1 was collected for the purpose of flushing out the nostril and removing any excess TE that had accumulated prior to the experimental session.

D. SYMPTOM SCORES

Clinical symptom scores were calculated as the sum of subjective symptom ratings for the first five items on the SSS form (runny nose, blocked nose, itchy nose, itchy palate, and watery eyes). Since the time-course for clinical responses varies between individuals,[33] the pre-challenge SSS was subtracted from the peak post-challenge SSS (i.e. either 5 minutes or 15 minutes post-challenge) to determine differences in SSS before and after challenge.

IV. RESULTS

Two subjects were excluded from the study after initial enrollment because they developed upper respiratory tract infections prior to the final experimental session. One other subject withdrew from the study. Therefore Groups 1, 2, and 3 included nine subjects each. Data from these subjects only were analysed.

A. TE ACTIVITY

TE activity scores (mean peak post-challenge value minus mean pre-challenge value) were transformed by adding 1605 to each score, to avoid negative overall scores. Statistical analyses were performed on transformed data. Application of Bartlett's[1] test for Homogeneity of Variance revealed a marked heterogeneity of variance between groups for TE activity on all days (x^2 = 24.91, 15.22, and 31.42, d.f.=2, $p < 0.05$ for CD1, CD2, and test day respectively. Multiple comparisons among variances on CD1[34] showed that all group variances were significantly different from each other ($p < 0.05$). Groups contributed to the overall variance in the following order: Group 1 > Group 3 > Group 2. The same sequence was observed on CD2, except that the Group 1 variance was not significantly different from the variance contributed by Group 3. On test day a similar pattern of variances occurred, except that Group 1 contributed significantly more variance than either group 2 or Group 3 ($p < 0.05$), and there was no significant difference between the variances of Group 2 and 3.

Since the assumption of homogeneity of variance was violated, nonparametric statistics were used to analyse TE activity. A Kruskal-Wallace analysis of variance showed that the difference in TE activity on CD1 between groups was significant (x^2 = 8.903, d.f=2, $p < 0.05$). Nonparametric multiple comparisons[35] revealed that TE activity was greater in Groups 1 and 3 compared with Group 2 ($p < 0.05$) (Fig.1). A similar conclusion was reached for TE activity on CD2 (x^2 = 14.098, d.f.=2, $p < 0.001$) (Fig.1). Therefore, comparison of TE activity distinguished between groups challenged with allergen (Groups 1 and 3) and control Group 2 (given PBS) on both conditioning days. On test day, a significant difference was also apparent in TE activity between groups (χ^2 = 6.321, d.f.=2, p<0.05). Application of Nemenyi's[35] nonparametric multiple comparisons revealed that enzyme activity was greater in Group 3 compared with Group 2 (p<0.05). Unlike the results for CD1 and CD2, however, the difference in TE activity between Group 1 and Group 2 on test day failed to reach significance (Fig.1). The large variance contributed by Group 1 TE activity on test day discussed above may account for this lack of significance.

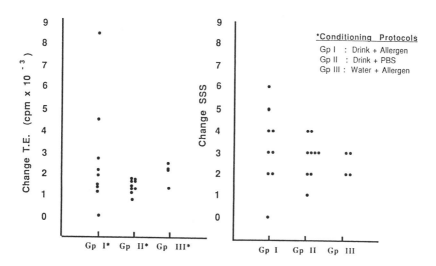

Figure 1. Changes in TE activity and subjective symptom score (SSS) on conditioning days and test day for each subject (expressed as peak post-challenge data minus mean pre-challenge data.

Together, these results suggest that the conditioning protocol employed in this study had effected TE release from mucosal mast cells on test day in Group 3, indicating that generalised conditioning had occurred i.e. conditioning to aspects of the environment other than the controlled CS *per se*.

The lack of overall increased TE activity on test day seen in Group 1 subjects implied that incorporation of the novel drink as a CS into the experimental protocol affected the generalised conditioned release of TE. However, the large variance contributed by Group 1 on test day indicated that the drink affected individuals differently. Inspection of individual data points shows that on test day some subjects had extremely high scores compared with control Group 2, while others had scores which were similar to Group 2 scores (Fig.1). This finding suggests that the novel drink may have a bi-modal effect on conditioning of AR and explains why no overall difference in TE values was reached. It was noted, however, that the presence of both the allergen challenge and the novel drink CS were necessary to effect this heterogeneity of variance since it did not occur if the drink had not previously been paired with the UCS.

B. SUBJECTIVE SYMPTOM SCORES

SSS scores were transformed by adding 2 to every score to avoid negative scores after subtracting the pre-challenge value from the highest post-challenge value. Statistical analyses were performed on transformed data. Non-pararametric statistics were employed to analyse SSS data because scores consisted of ordinal data. A Kruskal-Wallace analysis of variance showed that significant inter-group differences existed for CD1 and CD2 (χ^2 = 12.18 and χ^2 = 16.13 respectively, d.f.=2, p<0.01). These results indicate that SSS distinguished between groups challenged with allergen (Groups 1 and 3) and control Group 2 challenged with PBS (Fig.2). On test day there were no significant inter-group differences in SSS, however, indicating that conditioning of allergic symptoms had not been effected in either Group 1 or Group 3.

V. DISCUSSION

Conditioned release of nasal mucosal mast cell mediators in type 1 allergic reactions in humans has not been reported in the literature although individual case studies have suggested that conditioning of allergic symptoms is possible in certain individuals.[23-25] Several animal studies, however, have shown that conditioned release of mast cell mediators can be effected under controlled conditions.[27,28,36] In this study, conditioning of AR as measured by TE activity (an indicator of mast cell mediator release) and SSS (a subjective indicator of allergic symptoms) was attempted in allergic individuals in a controlled environment. It was expected that of the two, the measure TE activity would be a more reliable and sensitive indicator of AR because of its greater objectivity than the SSS scale values. Although both indicators readily discriminated subjects who had been challenged with allergen from those who received only PBS on CD1 and CD2, TE activity alone detected AR on test day. Therefore, the TE assay is superior for future studies on conditioning of AR.

The results indicated that a form of generalised conditioning had been effected in Group 3. It appears that a particular uncontrolled cue or set of cues acting as conditioning stimuli implicit in the experimental protocol became associated with allergen (the UCS) during the conditioning days so that on re-exposure to these CS factors, increased TE activity occurred.

There are many potential associative cues in this regard. For example, features of the experimenter, other object(s) in the room, or procedures performed during the experimental session may have acted as conditioning stimuli. In addition, subjective expectation of an allergic reaction may have resulted from the experimenter's statement that the subject would be challenged with allergen
followed by the suggestion that symptoms of hay fever may be experienced. The expectation would have been strengthened after symptoms of allergy were actually experienced upon

allergen challenge on CD1 and reinforced when the experience was repeated on CD2. Subjective expectation may be classed as a CS because the suggestion of an allergic reaction was paired with allergen challenge on conditioning days i.e. associative learning was involved.

It is important to note that the the presence of the UCS on conditioning days was necessary for the release of TE on test day. Therefore the suggestion of an allergic reaction *per se* was not sufficient to elicit AR as indicated by the lack of raised TE activity shown by Group 2 subjects on any day. The necessity of the presence of both CS and UCS for release of TE to be effected supports the model for conditioned AR.

The relative importance of subjective expectation compared with unspecified conditioning stimuli implicit in the experimental design cannot be assessed. In future studies, however, the effect of expectation could be separated from the effects of other experimental stimuli, by including a control group for each of Groups 1, 2 and 3 to whom nothing would be said about the impending allergen challenge or its likely allergic effects.

The conditioned-response model outlined above may provide a more specific explanation for many well documented accounts of placebo phenomena, i.e. the association of the administration of inert substances with therapeutic responses. For example the presence of a syringe or the ingestion of a pill associated with a particular drug therapy can function as conditioning stimuli to re-enlist the effects of the drug when it is replaced by a neutral substance.[37-39]

The generalised conditioned effect described above for Group 3 subjects appears to have been modified by the treatment experienced by Group 1 subjects. There was no difference between the responses of Group 1 and Group 3 on conditioning days. On test day, however, Group 1, unlike Group 3, failed to show a conditioned TE activity response. It was noted that Group 1 subjects exhibited a greater degree of variability among TE scores compared with Group 3. Since the only difference between these groups was the incorporation of the novel flavoured drink in Group 1 compared with tap water in Group 3, it appears that the drink was the critical factor eliciting this variability and ultimately in determining whether or not conditioning of TE release would be effected.

Inspection of individual data points suggests that the novel drink had a bi-modal effect on the expression of conditioned AR (Fig.1). In some individuals, the drink appeared to function synergistically as a compound CS with the associatory cues discussed above. This compound CS elicited conditioned effects which were greater than those attributed to the generalised cues alone. This explanation accounts for the extremely high TE values which characterised some Group 1 individuals.

On the other hand, in other individuals, the drink appeared to counteract the effects of the generalised cues in producing conditioned AR. This explanation accounts for the TE values of Group 1 individuals who showed similar scores to Group 2 control individuals. It should be noted that the bi-modal effect of the novel drink on conditioning of AR was only apparent if its consumption was followed by allergen challenge since the drink alone produced no such effect. However, the incorporation of an additional control Group which received water + PBS on both conditioning and test days would isolate any effects caused by the drink alone.

One interpretation of the neutralising effect the novel drink exerted on conditioned AR in some individuals may be attributed to a placebo effect which functioned antagonistically to the generalised conditioned effect described above. It is possible that those Group 1 subjects who did not exhibit raised TE activity on test day may have regarded the novel drink as a medication with potential to alleviate AR. Such subjects would not have expected to experience allergic symptoms after allergen challenge.

This expectation was possible because many subjects were recruited as the result of advertising which stated that the study was concerned with "alternative" treatments for hay fever and allergic rhinitis. In addition, the novel drink was mentioned in the consent form. Therefore, expectations about allergy-reducing properties of the drink may have been generated prior to participation in the experiment or shortly after commencement. It is proposed that in certain Group 1 individuals, this expectation over-rode other cues which promoted conditioning of AR. This interpretation is supported by another study which showed that the inhalation of a placebo substance by asthmatics reversed suggested bronchoconstrictive responses.[40]

Individual differences to the placebo effect are well documented which explains why the the novel drink appeared to exert differential effects on Group 1 subjects.[39,41-43] Future studies on the interactions of sex, age, intellectual status, and psychological variables such as state and trait anxiety, levels of overall stress, locus of control, and susceptibility to suggestion may aid in partitioning out factors which are contributing to the conditioning of AR and those which are opposing this effect.

In summary, the results of this experiment have implicated roles for generalised conditioning cues, specific conditioning cues, subjective expectations and the placebo effect in the onset of AR. The relative importance of each factor is subject to further investigations. However, it appears that associative learning can trigger the release of mucosal mast cell mediators, which are normally released in allergic rhinitis only after allergen exposure. This study therefore contributes to the growing body of research which implicates interactions between the CNS and the immune system. More specifically, the study has indicated that psychological manipulations may be beneficial in the management of allergic disorders in certain individuals.

VI. ACKNOWLEDGEMENTS

This work was supported by grants from the National Health and Medical Research Concil of Australia and the Rebecca L. Cooper Medical Research Foundation.

VII. REFERENCES

1.   Bartlett, M.S., Properties of sufficiency and statistical tests, *Proc.R.Soc.Lond.[A].]*, 160, 1, 1937.
2.   Solomon, G.F. and Moos, R.H., Emotions, immunity and disease,

Arch.Gen.Psychiatry, 11, 657, 1964.

3. Shavit, Y., Lewis, J.W., Terman, G.W., Gale, R.P. and Liebeskind, J.C., Opioid peptides mediate the suppressive effect of stress on natural killer cell cytotoxicity, *Science*, 223, 188, 1984.

4. Kraut, R.P. and Greenberg, A.H., Effects of endogenous and exogenous opioids on splenic natural killer cell activity, *Nat.Immun.Cell Growth Regul.*, 5, 28, 1986.

5. Kusnecov, A.W., Husband, A.J., King, M.G., Pang, G. and Smith, R., In vivo effects of B endorphin on lymphocyte proliferation and interleukin 2 production, *Brain Behav.Immun.*, 1, 88, 1987.

6. Kusnecov, A.W., Husband, A.J., King, M.G. and Smith, R., Modulation of mitogen-induced spleen cell proliferation and the antibody-forming cell response by beta-endorphin in vivo, *Peptides*, 10, 473, 1989.

7. Besedovsky, H.O., del Rey, A.E. and Sorkin, E., Immune-neuroendocrine interactions, *J.Immunol.(Suppl.)*, 135, 750s, 1985.

8. del Rey, A.E., Besedovsky, H.O., Sorkin, E. and Dinarello, C.A., Interleukin-1 and glucocorticoid hormones integrate an immunoregulatory feedback circuit, *Ann.N.Y.Acad.Sci.*, 496, 85, 1987.

9. Harbour-McMenamin, D., Smith, E.M. and Blalock, J.E., Bacterial lipopolysaccharide induction of leukocyte-derived corticotrophin and endorphins, *Infect.Immun.*, 48, 813, 1985.

10. Gorczynski, R.M., Macrae, S. and Kennedy, M., Conditioned immune response associated with allogeneic skin grafts in mice, *J.Immunol.*, 129, 704, 1982.

11. Ghanta, V.K., Hiramoto, R.N., Solvason, H.B. and Spector, N.H., Neural and environmental influences on neoplasia and conditioning of NK activity, *J.Immunol.*, S135, 848s, 1985.

12. Bovbjerg, D., Cohen, N. and Ader, R., Behaviorally conditioned enhancement of delayed-type hypersensitivity in the mouse, *Brain Behav.Immun.*, 1, 64, 1987.

13. Husband, A.J., King, M.G. and Brown, R., Behaviourally conditioned modification of T cell subset ratios in rats, *Immunol.Lett.*, 14, 91, 1987.

14. Ader, R. and Cohen, N., Behaviorally conditioned immunosuppression, *Psychosom.Med.*, 37, 333, 1975.

15. Neveu, R.J., Dantzer, R. and Le Moal, M., Behaviorally conditioned immunosuppression of mitogen-induced lymphoproliferation and antibody production in mice, *Neurosci.Lett.*, 65, 293, 1986.

16. O'Reilly, C.A. and Exon, J.H., Cyclophosphamide-conditioned suppression of the natural killer cell response in rats, *Physiol.Behav.*, 37, 759, 1986.

17. Kusnecov, A.W., Husband, A.J. and King, M.G., Behaviourally conditioned suppression of mitogen-induced proliferation and immunoglobulin production: Effect of time span between conditioning and reexposure to the conditioning stimulus, *Brain Behav.Immun.*, 2, 198, 1988.

18. Pavlov, I.P., *Conditioned Reflexes*, Oxford University Press, London, 1927,

19. Ader, R. and Cohen, N., CNS-immune system interactions: Conditioning pehnomena, *Behav.Brain Sci.*, 8, 379, 1985.

20. Bernstein, I.L., Learned taste aversions in children receiving chemotherapy, *Science*, 200, 1302, 1978.

21. Morrow, G.R., Prevalence and correlates of anticipatory nausea and vomiting in chemotherapy patients, *J.Natl.Cancer Inst.*, 68, 585, 1981.

22. Kiecolt-Glaser, J.K. and Glaser, R., Psychological influences on immunity:

Implicaztions for AIDS, *Am.Psychol.*, 43, 892, 1988.

23. MacKenzie, J.N., The production of "rose asthma" by an artificial rose, *Am.J.Med.Sci.*, 91, 45, 1886.
24. Dekker, E. and Groen, J., Reproducible psychogenic attacks of asthma, *J.Psychosom.Res.*, 1, 58, 1956.
25. Dekker, E., Pelser, H.E. and Groen, J., Conditioning as a cause of asthmatic attacks, *J.Psychosom.Res.*, 2, 97, 1957.
26. Smith, G.R.J. and McDaniel, S.M., Psychologically mediated effect on the delayed hypersensitivity reaction to tuberculin in humans, *Psychosom.Med.*, 45, 65, 1983.
27. Russell, M., Dark, K.A., Cummins, R.W., Ellmann, G., Callaway, E. and Peeke, H.V.S., Learned histamine release, *Science*, 225, 733, 1984.
28. MacQueen, G., Marshall, J., Perdue, M., Siegel, S. and Bienenstock, J., Pavlovian conditioning of rat mucosal cells to secrete rat mast cell protease II, *Science*, 243, 83, 1989.
29. Linder, A., Symptom scores as measures of the severity of rhinitis, *Clin.Allergy*, 18, 29, 1988.
30. Naclerio, R.M., Meier, H.L., Kagey-Sobotka, A., Adkinson, N.F.J., Meyers, D.A., Norman, P.S. and Lichtenstein, L.M., Mediator release after nasal airway challenge with allergen, *Am.Rev.Resp.Dis.*, 128, 597, 1983.
31. Schwartz, L.B., Yuringer, J.W., Miller, J., Bokhari, R. and Dull, D., Time course of appearance and disappearance of human mast cell tryptase in the circulation after anaphylaxis, *J.Clin.Invest.*, 83, 1551, 1989.
32. Proud, D., Togias, A., Naclerio, R.M., Crush, S.A., Norman, P.S. and Lichtenstein, L.M., Kinins are generated in vivo following nasal airways challenge of allergic individuals with allergen, *J.Clin.Invest.*, 72, 1678, 1983.
33. Castells, M. and Schwazrtz, L.B., Tryptase levels in nasal lavage fluid as an indicator of the immediate allergic response, *J.Allergy Clin.Immunol.*, 82, 348, 1988.
34. Levy, K.J., Some multiple range tests for variances, *Ed.Psych.Meas.*, 35, 599, 1975.

35. Nemenyi, P., *Distribution-Free Multiple Comparisons*, State University of New York Press, Downstate Medical Center, New York, 1963,
36. Peeke, H.V.S., Dark, K., Ellman, G., McCurry, C. and Salfi, M., Prior stress and behaviourally conditioned histamine release, *Physiol.Behav.*, 39, 89, 1987.
37. Lang, W.J. and Rand, M.J., A placebo response as a conditioned reflex to glyceryl nitrate, *Med.J.Aust.*, 1, 912, 1969.
38. Wickramasekera, I., A conditioned response model of the placebo effect: Predictions from the model, *Biofeedback Self Regul.*, 5, 5, 1980.
39. Butler, C. and Steptoe, A., Placebo responses: An experimental study of psychophysiological processes in asthmatic volunteers, *Br.J.Clin.Psych.*, 25, 173, 1986.
40. Spector, S.L., Luparello, T.J., Kopetzky, M.T., Souhrada, J. and Kinsman, R.A., Response of asthmatics to methacholine and suggestion, *Am.Rev.Resp.Dis.*, 113, 43, 1976.
41. Liberman, R., An experimental study of the placebo response under three different situations of pain, *J.Psychatr.Res.*, 2, 233, 1964.
42. Kellogg, R. and Baron, R.S., Attribution theory, insomnia, and the reverse placebo effect: A reversal of Storm and Nisbett's findings, *J.Pers.Soc.Psychol.*, 32, 231, 1975.

43.   Neild, J.E. and Cameron, I.R., Bronchoconstriction in response to suggestion: Its prevention by an inhaled anticholinergic agent, *Br.Med.J.*, 290, 674, 1985.

THERMOREGULATION: MODULATION OF BODY TEMPERATURE THROUGH BEHAVIOURAL CONDITIONING

Diane F. Bull, Richard Brown, Maurice G. King, Alan J. Husband[a], and
H.Peter Pfister

Department of Psychology and [a]Faculty of Medicine
The University of Newcastle, NSW, 2308, Australia

I. ABSTRACT

Recent investigations have demonstrated the susceptibility of various components of the immune system to behavioural conditioning using a conditioned taste aversion (CTA) paradigm. Work done in this laboratory has found the effects of several pyretic and anti-pyretic substances that, when incorporated as unconditioned stimuli (UCS) in CTA paradigms, can be re-enlisted upon re-exposure to the conditioned stimuli (CS). Using saccharin as the CS, these differential effects on body temperature were re-enlisted upon re-exposure to saccharin alone 7 days after conditioning. In this paper three experiments are described in which lipopolysaccharide (LPS), Lithium chloride (LiCl), and α-Melanocyte-stimulating hormone (MSH) are paired with a novel tasting saccharin solution to elicit conditioned pyretic or anti-pyretic responses. The antipyretic effects of MSH and LiCl and the pyretic effect of LPS were found to be significantly conditionable. The conditioning of pyretic/ antipyretic responses demonstrates that body temperature is subject to behavioural conditioning effects. Since body temperature changes often occur in association with immune responses, these findings may have implications to behavioural conditioning of immunity, the outcome of which may reflect the indirect effects on immunity of inadvertent conditioning of thermoregulatory changes.

II. INTRODUCTION

Reports from this and other laboratories have documented the susceptibility of various components of the immune system to behavioural conditioning using a taste aversion paradigm.[1-3] This technique involves the pairing of a salient conditioned stimulus (CS), such as a novel taste in drinking water, with a potent immunomodulatory agent, which acts as an unconditioned stimulus (UCS). With subsequent presentation of the CS, the subject exhibits conditioned taste aversion which is indexed empirically by a reduction in the consumption of the novel tasting substance. Concomitantly, the CS alone also elicits certain changes in the immune response which were previously attributable only to the stimulus.

One component of the immune response that has been found to respond to a conditioned stimulus is thermoregulation.[4,5] The fever response to antigen stimulation is an important part of the organism's defence. The initiating step in most immune responses involves antigen uptake by macrophages resulting in macrophage activation and Interleukin-1 (IL-1) production with a concomitant elevation in body temperature, the effect of which is to enhance IL-1 dependent immune mechanisms.[6,7]

Either increased or decreased body temperatures may be beneficial to the immune response, depending upon which activity is deemed desirable to enhance. For instance, increases in temperature dramatically augment the action of IL-1 on T-cell proliferative responses,[7] and cellular activity such as membrane resistance and potassium conductivity is highly temperature sensitive, with membrane potential having a positive temperature co-efficient which increases and temperature increases. Conversely, the amplitude and duration of the action potential are enhanced at lower temperatures,[8] and importantly the activity of natural killer cells, a vital part of the immune defence, is substantially reduced at febrile temperatures.[7]

The data in this paper bring together findings published elsewhere[4,9] which indicate the extent to which the febrile component of an immune response may be regulated by behavioural conditioning. In Experiment 1 LPS was investigated as a model for immune system activation to explore the extent to which this early phase of the immune response pathway is conditionable. For comparison, LiCl was used in Experiment 2 as an alternative UCS since this substance has been shown to induce powerful taste aversion behavioural responses[10] but is not a recognised pyrogen. Following on from the first two experiments it was decided to investigate whether a decrease in temperature from a febrile state was possible. In Experiment 3 the effect of MSH, an endogenous antipyretic,[11] and aspirin on a LPS induced fever was examined within the CTA paradigm. Both MSH and aspirin have been shown to reduce fever without affecting normal body temperature.[12]

The results reported here describe the conditioned changes in body temperature which occur in animals subjected to these protocols and demonstrate that for each of the unconditioned stimuli the responses following re-exposure to the CS alone were similar in direction and kinetics, although reduced in magnitude, compared to that following the initial UCS exposure.

III. MATERIALS AND METHODS.

A total of 110 rats aged between 90 and 100 days at the start of the experiments were used. All rats were of the inbred Australian Albino Wistar strain. Those used in Experiments 1 and 3 were obtained from the Australian Atomic Energy Commission (AAEC), Lucas Heights, Australia, and those in Experiment 2 were bred at the University of Newcastle Central Animal House from AEEC stock. Animals were housed individually in standard mesh wire cages, external dimensions 14.5 x 20 x 26 cm, in air conditioned holding rooms with an ambient temperature of $22 \pm 1°C$. Standard laboratory food pellets and tap water were available *ad libitum* and a 12:12 light/dark cycle with lights on at 1800 h and off at 0600 h was maintained throughout the experiment.

After a 2 week acclimatisation period all rats were subjected to a habituation regime during which they were placed on a water deprivation schedule which allowed drinking for 15 min at 1000 h each day. A two bottle system was employed during this experiment.

Baseline consumption was determined and no outliers were observed. During the habituation phase, all rats were handled gently and rectal temperatures were taken at 1000 h daily to establish baseline temperature data and to accustom animals to the procedure. A Cole-Parmer 08402 microcomputer rectal thermometer with thermistor probe was used to record temperatures. The probe was inserted 2.5cm into the rectum and temperatures were read when the display had stabilised for 10 s after a 60 s period. The thermometer was accurate to 0.1° C. The lipopolysaccharide (LPS) used was from the *Eschericia coli* strain (026:B6 Difco) while MSH was supplied by Sigma Chemicals. Pyrogen-free 0.9% saline solution (SAL) and 300mg Aspirin (ASP) were also used.

After 7 days of habituation, rats were allocated at random to experimental groups (see Table 1). For Experiments 1 and 2 during the drinking period of day 7 one of the bottles contained the appropriate CS (either normal water or 0.1% saccharin in water). Immediately following the 15 min drinking period, each rat received an intraperitoneal injection of the relevent UCS (either LPS (l00ug/kg), or LiCl (50mg/kg) or pyrogen-free saline) in a dose volume of 1.0 ml. After a further 7 days all rats were re-exposed only to the relevant CS, again in a two bottle fashion, during the 15 min drinking period.

For Experiment 3, all animals underwent the same training regimen as for Experiments 1 and 2. On Day 7 the animals were randomly allocated to seven groups.

Table 1. Treatment groups for Experiments 1 and 2.

Group Designation	No. Rats	Conditioning Day		Test Day
		CS +	UCS	CS
Experiment 1				
SAC/LPS	10	Saccharin	LPS	Saccharin
WAT/LPS	4	Water	LPS	Water
SAC/SAL	4	Saccharin	Saline	Saccharin
WAT/SAL	4	Water	Water	Water
Experiment 2				
SAC/LiCl	8	Saccharin	LiCl	Saccharin
WAT/LiCl	8	Water	LiCl	Water
SAC/SAL	8	Saccharin	Saline	Saccharin
WAT/SAL	8	Water	Saline	Water

Table 2. Treatment groups for Experiment 3.

Group	Drug Protocol			
	Test Day 1		Test Day 8	
α-MSH/SAC	LPS;α-MSH/SAC	Sal;	/SAC	
α-MSH/WAT	LPS;α-MSH/WAT	Sal;	/WAT	
ASP/SAC	LPS;ASP/SAC	Sal;	/SAC	
ASP/WAT	LPS;ASP/WAT	Sal;	/WAT	
SAL/SAC	LPS;ASP/WAT	Sal;	/SAC	
SAL/WAT	LPS;SAL/WAT	Sal;	/WAT	
SAL/SAC	SAL;SAL/SAC	Sal;	/WAT	

Six of the groups were allocated to the drug condition (see Table 2) while the seventh served as an additional SAL control for the saccharin consumption comparison. On Day 7 one hour prior to the normal drinking time (0900 h) 6 of the 7 groups received a 1.0ml intraperitoneal injection of 100ug/kg LPS to induce fever. At 1000 h immediately following the drinking period with the bottles containing the appropriate CS all experimental animals received the UCS injection specific to their group: 40 μg/kg MSH, 300mg/kg ASP, or 1.0ml of 0.9% saline solution.

For all 3 experiments, fluid consumption from the bottle containing the UCS was recorded on the conditioning day (Day 7) and test day (Day 14) to determine whether taste aversion had been established. The rectal temperatures were monitored at hourly intervals for a 12 h penod following each CS exposure for all groups in all 3 expenments for conditioning day (Day 7) and re-exposure day (Day 14).

IV. RESULTS

EXPERIMENT 1

Fluid consumption on conditioning day (Day 7) and test day (Day 14) for rats in experiment 1 are shown in Figure 1. There was no significant difference between groups with respect to consumption on Day 7 but on Day 14 conditioned taste aversion was observed in the SAC+LPS group which consumed significantly less that the WAT+LPS control groups (t - 5.34; df - 12; $p < 0.0001$).

The mean rectal temperatures recorded in these rats on the conditioning and test days are shown in Figure 2. Baseline temperatures recorded daily at 1000 h over the 7 days preceding days showed little variation (37.01 $\pm$ 0.04°C, mean $\pm$ SE) and this value is recorded as the common 0h temperature in Figure 2. In groups injected with LPS, whether given in association with saccharin or water, there was a fall in temperature for 2 h after

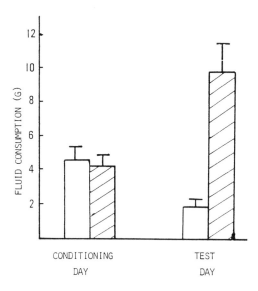

Figure 1. Consumption of saccharin in experimental (□ SAC+LPS) and control (▨ SAC+SAL) groups on conditioning day (Day 7) and test day (Day 14) in Experiment 1. Histograms represent mean values and vertical bars are standard errors. (Adapted from Bull *et al.*[4])

which mean temperatures rose to a peak above the normal temperature at 8h after injection. Rats injected with SAL displayed relatively constant temperatures for the first 3 h then a steady decline until 11 h after injection when the temperature began to rise again. This decline in temperature in saline control rats was associated with the approach and onset of the sleep period (lights on occurred at 7 h after injection. A repeated measures ANOVA revealed significant effects of Group ($F[3,18] - 42.51$, $p < 0.0001$), Time ($F[12,216] - 10.19$, $p < 0.0001$), and Group X Time ($F[36,216] - 47.70$, $p < 0.0001$). Post hoc analyses revealed significant differences between each of the LPS injected groups and the relevant SAL injected groups at both the hypothermic low point (2 h) and the hyperthermic peak (8 h). There was no significant difference between the SAC+LPS and the WAT+LPS groups in the mean temperature recorded at either 2 h or 8 h. Mean rectal temperatures recorded after CS re-exposure on test day (Day 14) indicated for all non-conditioned groups a pattern similar to that recorded for control groups on Day 7. In contrast, the SAC+LPS groups displayed a pattern which was similar in direction and kinetics to that observed following LPS injection on conditioning day with relative hypothermia lasting until 5 h after CS re-exposure, followed by a rise in temperature reaching a peak at 7 h. ANOVA revealed no significant Group effect, but significant effects for Time ($F[12,180] - 66.48$, $p < 0.0001$), and Group X Time ($F[24,180] - 9.23$ $p < 0.0001$). Post hoc comparisons indicated a significant difference between the SAC+LPS and WAT+LPS groups at 5 h, 7h, and 9 h after CS re-exposure.

EXPERIMENT 2

When LiCl was substituted for LPS in an identical experimental design all groups consumed similar amounts at first CS exposure on Day 7 but taste aversion was again observed only in the conditioned group (SAC+LiCl) at CS re-exposure on test day (Figure 3) with significantly less UCS Consumption recorded than for the WAT+LiCl group (t = 8.67; df = 14; p< 0.0001).

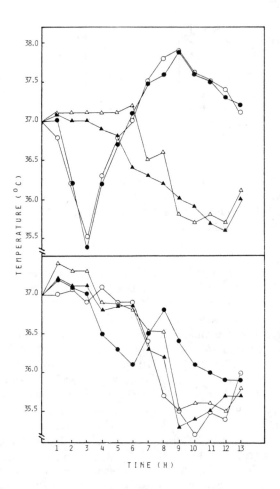

Figure 2. Mean rectal temperatures recorded in Experiment 1 on conditioning day (Day 7) and test day (Day 14) for SAC/SAL (▲-▲), WAT/SAL (△-△), SAC/LPS (●-●) and WAT/LPS (○-○) groups. (Adapted from Bull *et al.*[4])

Mean rectal temperatures for this experiment are shown in Figure 4. As in Experiment 1, baseline temperatures at 1000 h over the 7 days preceding conditioning and test days (36.97 $\pm$ 0.02°C, mean $\pm$ SE) was used as the common 0 h temperature. Rats injected with LiCl, whether paired with water or saccharin, displayed hypothermia reaching the lowest point at 2 h after injection and rising thereafter but never exceeding the mean temperatures recorded in saline control groups, returning to normal by 10 h. As in Experiment 1, saline controls showed no change in temperature during the early part of the recording period but a fall in temperature occurred towards the end of the period. This fall in temperature, representing the normal diurnal variation, was not as great as in the saline control groups in Experiment 1. ANOVA revealed significant effects of Group ($F[2,21]$ - 61.02, $p < 0.0001$), Time ($F[11,231]$ - 44.13, $p < 0.0001$) and Group X Time ($F[22,231]$ - 43.28, $p < 0.0001$). Post hoc comparisons revealed significant diffferences between each of the LiCl-injected groups and the complementary saline controls at 2 h after injection and CS exposure ($p = < .0001$). The SAC+LiCl and WAT+LiCl groups did not differ significantly at this time.

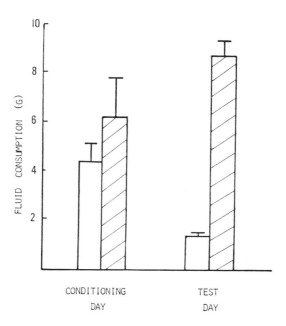

Figure 3.   Consumption of saccharin in experimental (☐ SAC+LiCl) and control (▨ SAC+SAL) groups on conditioning day (Day 7) and test day (Day 14) in Experiment 2. Histograms represent mean values and vertical bars are standard errors. (Adapted from Bull *et al.*[4])

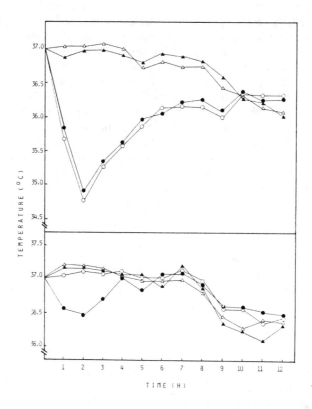

Figure 4. Mean rectal temperatures recorded in Experiment 2 on conditioning day (Day 7) and test day (Day 14) for SAC/SAL (▲-▲), WAT/SAL (△-△), SAC/LPS (●-●) and WAT/LPS (○-○) groups. (Adapted from Bull *et al*.[4])

After CS re-exposure on the test day (Day 14) the mean rectal temperature of all groups except the conditioned group (SAC+LiCl) remained unchanged initially but displayed a decline similar to that observed on Day 7 towards the end of the measurement period. In contrast, in the SAC+LiCl a fall in temperature was recorded during the first 2 h after CS re-exposure, but by 4 h and until the end of the recording period their temperature was not different from controls. ANOVA revealed significant effects for Time (F[11,231] - 44.6, p<0.0001), and Group X Time (F[22,231] - 6.83, p<0.0001) but there was no significant Group effect. Post hoc comparison at the 2 h time point for SAC+LiCl versus WAT+LiCl was significant (p= <.0001).

EXPERIMENT 3
The ANOVA performed on the data of test day (Day 7) revealed a significant difference between the 3 drug groups (MSH, ASP, and SAL) (F[2,42] - 2105.48, p<0.0001). The analysis showed that there was no significant difference in body temperature of animals

which were given tap water or saccharin as the CS (F[1,42] - .084, NS). There was a significant interaction between Drug X Time (F[18,378] - 483.85, p < 0.0001). Post hoc comparisons of the Drug X Time interaction revealed that for time t0, t1, t2, or t3 there was

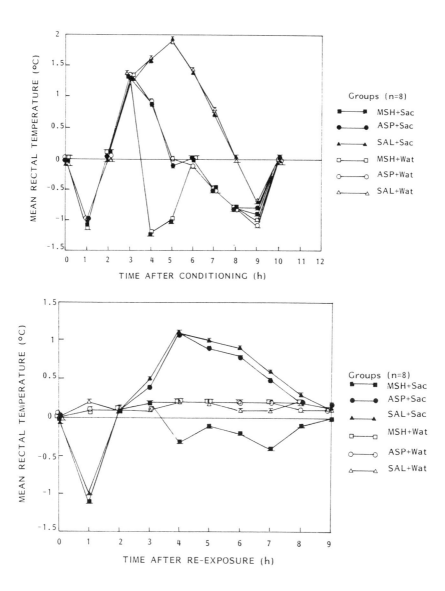

Figure 5. Mean rectal temperatures recorded in Experiment 3 on conditioning day (Day 7) (top panel) and test day (Day 14) (bottom panel). (Adapted from Bull *et al.*[9])

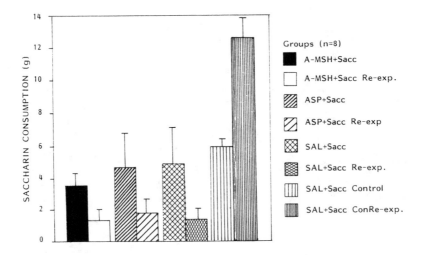

Figure 6. Consumption of saccharin for all groups on conditioning day (Day 7) and test day (Day 14). (Adapted from Bull *et al.*[9])

no significant difference of rectal temperature observed between the groups. At time t4 and t5, the rectal temperature of both MSH groups were significantly (p < .01) lower than that of both the ASP groups and the SAL groups, while the means of the ASP groups were also lower than the SAL groups (p < .01). The rectal temperatures for both the MSH and ASP groups were significantly lower than that of the SAL groups for time t6, t7, and t8 (p < .01), the previously observed significant differences between these two groups is, however, no longer observed at the time points. At time t9, no significant difference were observed in the rectal temperature of any of the groups.

The ANOVA performed on the day of re-exposure day (Day 14) revealed a significant main effect of the CS variable (F[1,42] - 16.03, p < 0.0002). Figure 5 indicates that there are significant differences between the groups re-exposed to saccharin and those re-exposed to water. In addition, the ANOVA revealed a significant Drug X Drink X Time interaction (F[18,379] - 81.76, p < 0.0001) effect. As can be seen from Figure 5, Post hoc comparisom confirmed that the significant (p < .01) interaction was due first to the lower rectal temperatures at time tl of the SAC+MSH, SAC+ASP, and SAC+SAL groups when compared to the rectal temperatures of the 3 water control groups. This decline in temperature was reversed for the SAC+ASP and SAC+SAL groups at time t3, t4, tS, t6, t7, and t8, being significantly (p < .01) elevated compared to the respective water control groups. The SAC+MSH and SAC+SAL groups displayed significantly (p < .Ol) reduced rectal temperatures at time t4, tS, t6, t7, and t8.

ANOVA performed on the saccharin consumption for the three groups revealed a significant (see Figure 6) Drug X Drink interaction (F[3,281] - 29.35, p < 0.0001). Post hoc comparison of the significant interaction demonstrated that there was a significant (p < .01) difference between the data obtained on re-exposure day (Day 14) of the SAC+SAL control group and the 3 experimental groups. The consumption of saccharin on re-exposure of the control groups was significantly higher (p < .01) than each of the other three groups. All 3 experimental groups drank significantly less on re-exposure day (Day 14) than they did on exposure day (Day 7) (p < .01), whereas the SAC+SAL control group drank significantly more on re-exposure day (Day 14) than they did on exposure day (Day 7) (p < .01).

V. DISCUSSION

These results demonstrate that in animals which have been treated with a UCS which modifies body temperature given in paired association with a CS, display taste aversion on CS re-exposure and a re-enlistment of the temperature changes associated with the acute response to injection in both direction and kinetics. The conditioned rise in body temperature by LPS in Experiment 1 is, although significant, smaller in magnitude when compared to the original pharmacological effect on Day 7. Conversely, the reduction in body temperature due to the conditioned MSH effect on test Day 14 in Experiment 3 is greater in magnitude when compared to the MSH effect obtained on Day 7.

Interestingly, aspirin which showed a modest anti-pyretic effect following LPS injection on Day 7 of Experiment 3 (see Figure 5) was not at all effective 7 days later on Day 14. From Figure 5, it is evident that the ASP group did not differ from the control SAL group, suggesting a qualitative difference in the action of ASP and MSH. This finding supports previous reports demonstrating that MSH and aspirin differ in their central mechanism of antipyresis.[13]

Both the acute and conditioned responses to LPS in all 3 experiments occurred in a biphasic manner; hypothermia followed by hyperthermia. The hyperthermic response to LPS is well documented and is known to be mediated by macrophage activation resulting in release of the cytokine Interleukin-1 (IL-1),[14] which acts upon the brainstem and anterior hypothalamus to alter the temperature regulatory mechanism.[15] The biphasic nature of the response to LPS appears to be a profile which is peculiar to rats[16] and some avian species[17,18] and is analogous to the temperature response to morphine injection reported by Gunne.[19] This suggests that these drugs might act on multiple pathways. The mechanisms producing the transient hypothermia which preceded this response are not clear but may reflect perturbation of a different physiologic pathway to that inducing the fever, perhaps the same pathway which was activated by the LiCl injection in Experiment 2. We suggest that whereas an LPS-induced fever is driven by lymphomyeloid activation, LiCl induced hypothermia and the initial hypothermia following LPS injection may represent a stress-driven response.

LiCl was chosen for Experiment 2 as an alternative UCS to provide a conditioning control, on the expectation that it would be neutral with respect to temperature effects although capable of inducing strong taste aversion behavioural conditioning. The hypothermia recorded as an acute response to LiCl was unexpected and to our knowledge has not been reported previously. A retrospective literature review yielded few reports where temperature change has been measured following LiCl administration.

The conditioned responses recorded for UCS substances in all 3 experiments represented accurate re-enlistment of the acute effects of the three drugs. This is in contrast to the paradoxical or compensatory conditioning of body temperatures reported by Dyck *et al*[20] using multiple cued injections of Poly I:C in a classical conditioning model. In those experiments the conditioned response provoked a temperature change in a direction opposite to the induced by the UCS. There are potentially two explanations for the apparent conflict between these date and the experiments reported in the present paper. Eikelboom and Stewart[12] have argued that in a system subject to negative feedback control, such as thermoregulation, the direction on the conditioned response is determined by whether the drug is acting on the afferent or efferent arm of the feedback loop. The response to drugs that act on the afferent arm will become the unconditioned response, and the conditioned response will then be in the same direction as the drug effect; drugs which act on the efferent arm will promote conditioning of the homeostatic compensatory response which will become the unconditioned response and the re-enlisted conditioned response will then oppose the original actions of the drug.

If the conditioned thermomodulation observed in these experiments are mediated by IL-1 release, then the experimental model will allow investigation of the hypothesis that the production of this cytokine, a key component in the initiation of an immune response, is a conditionable event. If this is the case, the present studies demonstrate that individual soluble factors may be conditionable, thus greatly simplilying immune conditioning paradigms and allowing a much clearer analysis of the factors involved. Subsequent studies examining the response of IL-1 serum levels as a function of taste pairing conditioning may add further support to this hypothesis.

VI. REFERENCES

1.   Ader, R. and Cohen, N., Behaviourally conditioned immuno-suppression, *Psychometr.Med.*, 37, 333, 1982.

2.   Husband, A.J., King, M.G. and Brown, R., Behaviourally conditioned modification of T cell subset ratios in rats, *Immunol.Lett.*, 14, 91, 1987.

3.   Kusnecov, A.W., Sivyer, M., King, M.G., Husband, A.J., Cripps, A.W. and Clancy, R.L., Behaviorally conditioned suppression of the immune response by antilymphocyte serum, *J.Immunol.*, 130, 2117, 1983.

4.   Bull, D.F., Brown, R., King, M.G. and Husband, A.J., Modulation of body temperature through taste aversion conditioning, *Physiol.Behav.*, 1991.(In Press)

5.   Farrar, W.L., Kilian, P.L., Ruff, M.R., Hill, J.M. and Pert, C.B., Visualization and characterization of interleukin-1 receptors in brain, *J.Immunol.*, 139, 459, 1987.

6.   Atkins, E., Fever: the old and the new, *J.Infect.Dis.*, 149, 339, 1984.

7.   Dinarello, C.A., Interleukin-1 and the pathogenesis of the acute-phase response, *New Eng.J.Med.*, 311, 1413, 1984.

8.   Gagge, A.P. and Stolwijk, J.A.J., *Physiological and Behavioural Temperature*

Regulation, Charles C. Thomas, Illinois, 1970.

9. Bull, D.F., King, M.G., Pfister, H.P. and Singer, G., Alpha-melanocyte-stimulating hormone conditioned suppression of a lipopolysaccharide-induced fever, *Peptides*, 111, 1027, 1990.

10. Alizadeh, H., Urban, J.F., Katona, I.M. and Finkelman, F.D., Cells containing IgE in the intestinal mucosa of mice infected with the nematode parasite Trichinella spiralis are predominantly of a mast cell lineage, *J.Immunol.*, 137, 2555, 1986.

11. Bell, R.E., Feng, J. and Lipton, J.M., Is the endogenous anti-pyretic neuropeptide MSH responsible for reduced fever in aged rabbits, *Peptides*, 8, 501, 1987.

12. Eikelboom, R. and Stewart, J., Conditioning of drug-induced physiological responses, *Psychol.Rev.*, 89, 507, 1982.

13. Scales, W.E. and Kluger, M.J., Effect of antipyretic drugs on circadian rhythm in body temperature of rats, *Am.J.Physiol.*, 253, 306, 1987.

14. Fontana, A., Weber, E. and Dayer, J.M., Synthesis of IL-1/ endogenous pyrogen in the brain of endotoxin- treated mice: a step in fever production, *J.Immunol.*, 133, 1697, 1984.

15. Rosendorff, C. and Mooney, J.J., Central nervous system sites of action of purified leukocyte pyrogen, *J.Physiol.*, 220, 995, 1978.

16. Krueger, J.M., Kubillus, S., Shoham, S. and Davenne, D., Enhancement of slow-wave sleep by endotoxin and lipid A, *J.Am.Physiol.Soc*, 10, 591, 1986.

17. Clark, W.G., Holdeman, M. and Lipton, J.M., Analysis of the anti-pyretic action of α-MSH hormone in rabbits, *J.Physiol.*, 359, 459, 1985.

18. Pittman, Q.J., Veale, W.L., Cockeram, A.W. and Cooper, K.E., Changes in body temperature produced by prostaglandins and pyrogens in the chicken, *Am.J.Physiol.*, 230, 1284, 1976.

19. Gunne, L.M., The temperature response in rats during acute and chronic morphine administration: a study of morphine tolerance, *Archs Int.Pharmacol.Ther.*, 129, 416, 1991.

20. Dyck, D.G., Osachuk, T.A.G. and Greenberg, A.H., Drug-induced (poly I:C) pyrexic responses: Congruence with a compensatory conditioning analysis, *Psychobiol.*, 17, 171, 1989.

ANTILYMPHOCYTE SERUM AND LITHIUM CHLORIDE AS A COMPOUND UNCONDITIONED STIMULUS FOR IMMUNOMODULATION

M. Gauci, D.F. Bull[a], M. Schedlowski[a], A.J. Husband and M.G. King[a]

Faculty of Medicine, and [a]Department of Psychology,
The University of Newcastle. NSW. 2308. Australia.

I. INTRODUCTION

It is well established that when rats are presented with a benign but novel gustatory conditioned stimulus (CS) followed immediately by an unconditioned stimulus (UCS) which induces an immunological response, both taste aversion and re-enlistment of the immunological effects of the UCS occur upon re-exposure to the CS alone. Such a response is an example of classical conditioning.[1,2]

In previous studies with rats, it was shown that when a weak saccharin solution (the CS) was paired with rabbit anti-rat lymphocyte serum (ALS) as the UCS, both taste aversion and conditioned immunosuppression were elicited when rats were later exposed to the saccharin solution alone.[3] Subsequent studies demonstrated that if LiCl, which has well documented taste aversion inducing properties,[4] was given with ALS as a compound UCS, the resultant conditioned behavioural response (taste aversion) was greater than that induced by either ALS or LiCl alone.[5] However, the effect of this compound UCS on conditioned immune parameters was not determined.

In conditioning studies, many reports have appeared in which LiCl has been used on the assumption that it is an immunologically neutral stimulus but elicits strong taste aversion because of its noxious side effects.[4] However, LiCl has been shown in some reports to induce immunoaugmentation[6,7] which can be re-enlisted as a conditioned response when LiCl is used as a UCS.[8,9] Indeed the effects of lithium on immune function appear to be most pronounced when immunity has been compromised[10,11] which is usually the case when an immunosuppressive UCS is used in conditioning experiments due to the residual effects of UCS administration.

The purpose of the study reported here was to determine whether LiCl could modify the conditioned immune response when given as a compound UCS with ALS. If LiCl is indeed immunologically neutral then the expectation would be that there would either be no change in the conditioned immune response or, if the magnitude of the conditioned behavioural response is correlated with that of the conditioned immune response, then more profound immunosuppression might be expected in view of the synergism observed previously in taste aversion when ALS and LiCl were given together.[5] On the other hand, in view of reports that LiCl may restore immune function in an immunosuppressed state, the level of conditioned immunosuppression may be reduced as a result of the immunoaugmenting effects of lithium in the presence of the residual effects of ALS treatment given at first CS/UCS exposure.

II. MATERIALS AND METHODS

A. ANIMALS

Ninety six male inbred Wistar rats aged 100-110 days were individually housed in hanging wire cages in soundproof cubicles with *ad libitum* access to food and water. A 12:12h light:dark cycle was maintained with lights on at 0600h.

B. ANTILYMPHOCYTE SERUM

ALS was prepared in two New Zealand white rabbits. Rabbits were given two intramuscular injections of mesenteric lymph node cells obtained from Wistar rats (1×10^7 cells per injection) 14 days apart followed 7 days later by two intravenous injections 7 days apart. The rabbits were bled weekly from the marginal ear vein on 4 consecutive weeks commencing 1 week after the last injection. They were exsanguinated by cardiac puncture on the fifth week. Sera were prepared, pooled and depleted of complement by heat inactivation at 56°C. Sera from 4 uninjected rabbits were pooled and heat inactivated to produce control normal rabbit serum (NRS). ALS and NRS were tested for cytotoxic activity against rat mesenteric lymph node cells using a chromium release assay.[12] At a dilution of 1:64, ALS produced 44% lysis of target cells while NRS produced only 3% lysis.

C. EXPERIMENTAL PROTOCOL

Following a 2 week acclimatisation period, rats were placed on an 8 day water restriction regimen during which water intake was restricted to one 15 min period commencing at 0600h each day. Rats were then allocated to one of 8 treatment groups (Table 1). On the eighth day (Day 0 of the conditioning protocol), rats were presented with either normal bottled water (Wat) or 0.2% saccharin in tap water (Sacc). Immediately following the 15 min drinking period, rats were injected with either 0.2ml ALS or 0.2ml NRS followed immediately by injection of either 0.3ml LiCl (50 mg/kg) or 0.3ml sterile phosphate buffered (pH7.4) saline (PBS). Animals were then returned to their cages. Six days after the conditioning day rats were again exposed to their respective CS (either Wat or Sac) and fluid intake was monitored by comparing bottle weights before and after drinking.

Rats were sacrificed by decapitation 24h after CS re-exposure (Day 7) and trunk blood collected into heparinised tubes and peripheral blood leukocytes counted using a haemocytometer. Spleens were removed and placed in PBS supplemented with 5% heat inactivated foetal calf serum (FCS), 0.2M L-glutamine and 0.5% mineral salts (Dulbecco). Spleen cell suspensions were prepared by chopping each spleen on a stainless steel sieve and pressing the tissue through the sieve into a petri dish containing 2ml supplemented PBS. The resulting suspensions were washed and leukocyte counts performed using a haemocytometer.

D. DATA ANALYSIS

Fluid consumption data for Days 0 and 6 were analysed using a two-way ANOVA with repeated measures for Day effects. Peripheral blood and spleen leukocyte counts on Day

TABLE 1. Experimental Protocol

Group	No. Rats	Day 0 CS	Day 0 UCS	Day 6 CS	Day 7
1.	12	Sacc	NRS + PBS	Sacc	Assay
2.	12	Sacc	NRS + LiCl	Sacc	Assay
3.	12	Wat	NRS + PBS	Wat	Assay
4.	12	Wat	NRS + LiCl	Wat	Assay
5.	12	Sacc	ALS + PBS	Sacc	Assay
6.	12	Sacc	ALS + LiCl	Sacc	Assay
7.	12	Wat	ALS + PBS	Wat	Assay
8.	12	Wat	ALS + LiCl	Wat	Assay

Sacc = saccharin 0.2% in drinking water; ALS = rabbit anti-rat lymphocyte serum; NRS = normal rabbit serum; PBS = phosphate buffered saline.

7 were analysed using one-way ANOVAs. Post hoc comparisons were performed where appropriate using the Fisher Least Significant Difference (LSD).[13]

III. RESULTS

A. BEHAVIOURAL RESPONSES

Fluid consumption on Day 0 and Day 6 for all treatment groups is shown in Fig 1. There were significant Group effects ($F(7,88) = 22.6$, $p < 0.0001$), Day effects ($F(1,88) = 56.0$, $p < 0.0001$) and Group X Day interaction effects ($F(7,88) = 19.75$, $p < 0.0001$). Post hoc comparisons for fluid consumption on Day 0 showed that there were no significant differences among the four groups receiving water or among the four groups receiving saccharin. However, the latter four groups consumed significantly less fluid than any group receiving water, demonstrating a neophobic response to the saccharin solution ($p < 0.01$). For groups receiving water there was no significant change in fluid consumption on Day 6 compared with Day 0 but on the other hand, the Sacc/NRS group drank significantly more fluid on Day 6 compared with Day 0 and was no different to that of any of the water groups, indicating that the neophobic response to saccharin had extinguished in this group. The Sacc/ALS group, however, continued to consume less fluid on re-exposure to saccharin

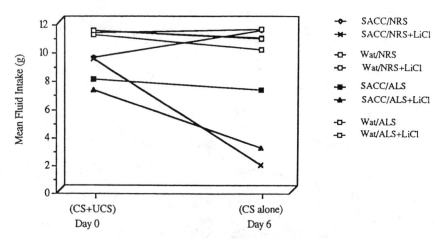

Figure 1.   Mean fluid consumption (g) on Day 0 (exposure to CS + UCS) and Day 6 (re-exposure to CS alone).

than the Wat/ALS group (p < 0.01). The Sacc/NRS + LiCl and Sacc/ALS + LiCl groups showed the greatest reduction in fluid consumption on Day 6, compared with the water groups (p < 0.01), also drinking significantly less fluid on Day 6 compared with Day 0 (p < 0.01).

These results reveal that taste aversion conditioning occurred in the Sacc/ALS, Sacc/ALS + LiCl, and Sacc/NRS + LiCl groups. The group receiving the compound UCS (i.e. ALS + LiCl) exhibited a greater degree of taste aversion than the group receiving ALS alone, but this was not significantly different from that displayed by the Sacc/NRS + LiCl group. This indicated that the contribution to taste aversion by LiCl and ALS were not additive and no synergism in behavioural response was apparent with the compound UCS.

B. IMMUNOLOGICAL RESPONSES
Peripheral blood leukocyte counts on Day 7 (Fig. 2) showed significant Group effects (F(7,87) = 8.119, p < 0.0001). Post hoc comparisons revealed that there were no significant differences in the mean leukocyte count for the Sacc/NRS group compared with the Wat/NRS group or the Sacc/NRS + LiCl group compared with the Wat/NRS + LiCl group. However the mean leukocyte count of the Sacc/ALS group was significantly lower than the Sacc/NRS group (p < 0.05) and likewise the Sacc/ALS + LiCl group mean leukocyte count was significantly lower than for the Sacc/NRS + LiCl group (p < 0.05). These data indicate that the lymphopaenia observed in the Sacc/ALS and Sacc/ALS + LiCl groups was not due to a conditioning effect since the Wat/ALS and Wat/ALS + LiCl groups displayed equivalent lymphopaenia, probably reflecting residual effects of the initial exposure to ALS.   The observation that the mean leukocyte count for the Wat/ALS + LiCl group was greater than that for the Wat/ALS group, although not statistically significant, was consistent with an antagonistic effect of LiCl on the immunosuppressive effects of ALS.

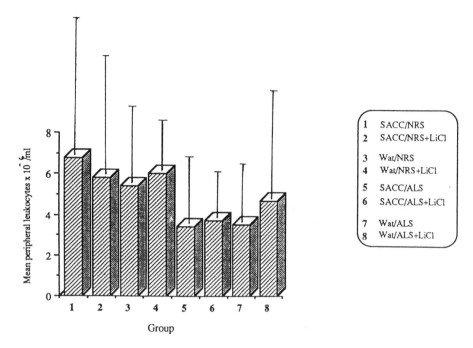

Figure 2.   Peripheral blood leukocyte count (mean $\pm$ SE) on Day 7.

Analysis of mean group spleen cell counts (Fig. 3) revealed significant Group effects $(F(7,87)=12.392, p<0.0001)$ and post hoc comparisons showed that the Sacc/ALS group had a lower mean spleen cell count than the Wat/ALS group $(p<0.05)$ indicating that the relative lymphopaenia occurred as a conditioned response. Conditioned immunosuppression was also apparent in the Sac/ALS + LiCl group which had a significantly lower spleen cell count than the Wat/ALS + LiCl group $(p<0.05)$. There was no significant difference in mean spleen cell count between the Sacc/ALS group and the Sacc/ALS + LiCl group, however, indicating a lack of synergistic effect on the conditioned immunological response when ALS and LiCl were administered as a compound UCS. Indeed the mean spleen cell count for the Sac/ALS + LiCl was marginally higher than for the Sacc/ALS group. It was also of interest to note that the residual immunosuppression due to the initial ALS treatment was reduced by LiCl since the Wat/ALS group had significantly fewer spleen cells recovered than the Wat/ALS + LiCl $(p<0.05)$. These data corroborate the findings for peripheral leukocyte counts in that the addition of LiCl appears to antagonise the immunosuppressive effects contributed by ALS.

IV. DISCUSSION

Analysis of the behavioural data presented here confirmed previous findings that both ALS and LiCl are effective in establishing taste aversion conditioning when administered as a UCS.[5] However, in these experiments, conditioned synergism in the behavioural response did not occur when these substances were given as a compound UCS, although LiCl was a

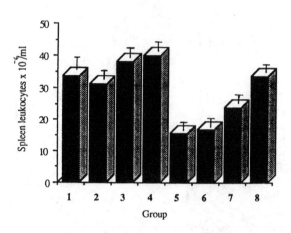
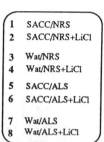

Figure 3.   Spleen cell count (mean ± SE) on Day 7.

more potent stimulant of taste aversion than was ALS, causing profound taste aversion whether given with ALS or NRS. A possible explanation for the failure to demonstrate synergism, in view of the previous report,[5] was that the ALS used in this experiment was lower in titre and therefore less potent than that used by Kusnecov *et al.*[5]

The immunological data showed that conditioned suppression of peripheral blood leukocyte numbers did not occur with either ALS or LiCl, whether administered singly or together as a compound UCS. However, conditioned suppression of spleen leukocyte numbers occurred in animals conditioned with Sacc/ALS, and in those conditioned with Sacc/ALS + LiCl, a finding which is consistent with a previous study showing that conditioned immunosuppression of mixed lymphocyte culture reactivity was achieved by this treatment using ALS as the UCS.[3]

The observation that the compound UCS (ALS + LiCl) in non-conditioned animals resulted in a reduced level of residual immunosuppression suggest that LiCl and ALS operate antagonistically and synergism in the conditioned immunological response would therefore not be a realistic expectation. The data therefore demonstrate that LiCl is not an immunologically neutral UCS and has effects on immunity which, in models of behaviourally conditioned immunosuppression, may operate to restore immunological function. This is supported by work reported elsewhere[10,11,14] showing that LiCl can restore immunological function in an immunocompromised individual. For example, treatment with lithium of patients with immunodeficiency diseases or autoimmune diseases results in improvement in the former condition and worsening in the latter.[10,11] *In vitro* studies have shown that lithium induces lymphocyte proliferation, rosette formation of T cells, and phagocytosis by macrophages.[7,10,14]

This augmented cellular immunity may be mediated by the inhibitory effects of lithium on the immunosuppressive properties of adenylate cyclase.[7,14] Therefore conclusions drawn from studies of behaviourally conditioned immunomodulation where LiCl is used as part of either the CS or UCS may require re-evaluation.

V. ACKNOWLEDGEMENTS

The work described in this paper was supported by grants from the National Health and Medical Research Council of Australia and the Australian Research Council.

VI. REFERENCES

1. Ader, R. and Cohen, N., Behaviorally conditioned immunosuppression, *Psychosom.Med.*, 37, 333, 1975.
2. Barker, L.M., Best, M.R. and Comjan, M., *Learning Mechanisms in Food Selection*, Baylor University Press, Waco, 1977.
3. Kusnecov, A.W., Sivyer, M., King, M.G., Husband, A.J., Cripps, A.W. and Clancy, R.L., Behaviorally conditioned suppression of the immune response by antilymphocyte serum, *J.Immunol.*, 130, 2117, 1983.
4. Riley, A.L. and Baril, L.L., Conditioned taste aversion: A bibliography, *Anim.Learn.Behav.*, (Suppl.)4, 1, 1991.
5. Kusnecov, A.W., King, M.G. and Husband, A.J., Synergism of a compound unconditioned stimulus in taste aversion conditioning, *Physiol.Behav.*, 39, 531, 1987.
6. Ader, R., Conditioned adrenocortical steroid elevation in the rat, *J.Comp.Physiol.Psychol.*, 90, 1156, 1976.
7. Shenkman, I., Borkowsky, W., Holzman, R.S. and Shopsin, B., Enhancement of lymphocyte and macrophage function in vitro by lithium chloride, *Clin.Immunol.Immunopathal.*, 10, 187, 1978.
8. Jenkins, P.E., Chadwick, R.A. and Nevin, J.A., Classically conditioned enhancement of antibody production, *Bull.Psychonomic Soc.*, 21, 485, 1983.
9. Hiramoto, R.H., Hiramoto, N.S., Solvason, H.B. and Ghanta, V.K., Regulation of natural immunity (NK activity) by conditioning, *Ann.N.Y.Acad.Sci.*, 496, 545, 1987.
10. Lieb, J., Lithium and immune function, *Med.Hypotheses*, 23, 73, 1987.
11. O'Connell, R.A., Leukocytosis during lithium carbonate treatment, *Int.Pharmacopsychiatry*, 4, 30, 1970.
12. Mishell, B.B. and Shiigi, S.M., *Selected methods in cellular immunology*, W.H.Freeman And Co., San Francisco, 1980.
13. Keppel, G., *Design and Analysis: A Researcher's Handbook*, 2nd ed., Prentice Hall, Englewood Cliffs, 1982.
14. Shenkman, L., Borkowsky, W. and Shopsin, B., Lithium as an immunologic agent, *Med.Hypotheses*, 6, 1, 1980.

III. Sleep and Biological Rhythms

RHYTHMICITY IN IMMUNITY AND IN FACTORS INFLUENCING IMMUNE RESPONSES

Martin S. Knapp

Renal Unit, Austin Hospital, Heidelberg. Vic. 3084. Australia.

I. ABSTRACT

There is now an extensive literature documenting rhythmicity in most body systems including the immune system and the central nervous system. There are large amplitude rhythms in many of the individual components of the immune system including, for example, many lymphocytes subsets. There are large amplitude rhythms demonstrated in immediate hypersensitivity and delayed hypersensitivity immune responses in vivo. There are rhythms in general of the hormone systems known to influence the immune system. The documented rhythms include circadian rhythms, around 24 hours, circaseptan rhythms around 7 days and circannual (seasonal) rhythms. Those involved in the study of behaviourial sciences in relation to immunology must take note of biological rhythmicity both in planning their experiments and in interpreting them. Rhythmicity must also be considered in field studies and in clinical practice.

II. INTRODUCTION

There is now an extensive literature to support the statement that in animals and man the magnitude of both humoral and cell-mediated responses is influenced by the body's biological rhythms. The amplitude of these predictable variations are not small.[1-5] Changes that take place in some immune responses due to their relationship to circadian or seasonal variations represent a change greater than is often achieved in the course of experiments studying other influences on immune responses, or when evaluating the effects of immuno-modulating therapy (Fig 1).

Many of those variables known to influence immune responses, or individual components of it, have been studied for rhythmic variations. Many of these show rhythmicity.[5-10] There are also many influences on the immune system now being studied that have not yet been adequately considered chronobiologically, among these are the many growth factors.[11,12] The control of the immune system is a subject that receives much attention, but is still poorly understood. It is not, therefore, surprising that what controls rhythms in the immune system is not known.

A failure to stabilise rhythms in experimental subjects, or to be consistent in the time of experiments, can greatly increase the variance and 'noise' when considering some immune responses. Studies should take into account the large variations in immunological events that are dependent on body time. Those who have not considered biological rhythmicity as a possible cause of variance in their test system, should consider the magnitude of change which is dependent only on the timing of a study. Change may be greater than what would be considered quite remarkable and exciting if induced by an intervention, for example by a new drug.

There is an extensive literature that establishes that the timing of an intervention, e.g., the administration of a medication, may have a marked influence on the effect of that intervention, both on the extent of desired effects and on the magnitude of undesired toxic effects.[6-10] Many agents used to influence immune responses have not been subjected to chronopharmacological study to evaluate the importance of timing, but when this has been done there are indicationg that the time of day or night when an immunomodulating medication is given may influence its effect and its toxicity.

Can techniques used by those with an interest in biological rhythmicity, and developed

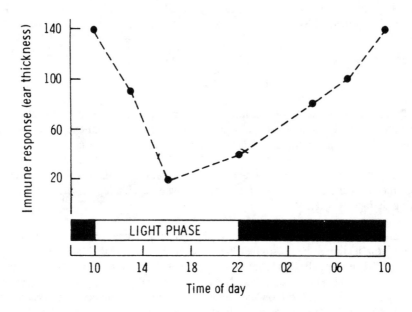

Figure 1 The time of administration of the antigen in relation to onset of light and dark in the 24 hour cycle influences the magnitude of a cell mediated immune response, as demonstrated by response to oxazolone in sensitised rats, Pownall and Knapp.[13]

to collect information on whether time is an influence on events, also assist the search for basic information about immune responses, or in the search for interactions between central nervous system function and aspects of behaviour? Studies into dissociationg of potential controlling systems while making observations on rhythmicity in the immune system or in controlling factors could progress understanding.

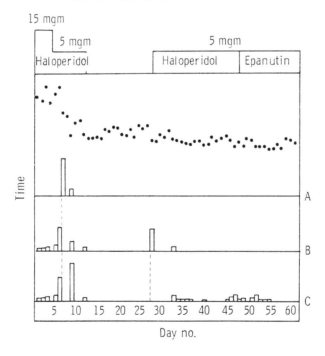

Figure 2. Retrospective change-point detection using Bayesian gamma-function analysis detecting change in performance when doing computer games in relation to Haloperidol and Epanutin administration.[14-16]

III. STATISTICAL METHODS

Statistical methods to establish the probability of any variationg observed being rhythmic phenomena, rather than being random 'noise', should be used in all studies. Rhythmic changes often approximate to sinusoidal, and analysis by the least squares method

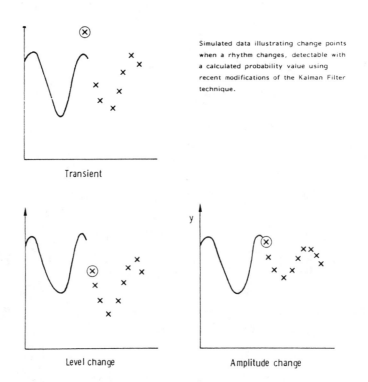

Figure 3. Prospective change-point detection in rhythmic data biotechnology.[14,17] On-line event detection should consider each new incoming item of information, and consider statistically if it could reasonably be expected from previous information on the patterns of information; taking into account the variability ('noise') in previous data. Change points with rhythm change, if instantaneous, may be indicated by as few as two points in a sequence of incoming information if in an unexpected, but anticipated, relationship to the previous pattern. Statistical methods that when first developed took no account of rhythmicity have now been modified to incorporate the reality that clinically important sequences of data are rhythmic (Knapp, Smith, Trimble, Pownall and Gordon[15]).

of analysis, sometimes referred to as the Cosinor method in chronobiological literature, are often adequate to establish rhythmicity, but do not exclude it when rhythmic change is non-sinusoidal or when there is inadequate data. In the summarised reports to follow, this method is most often used other than when stated. Standard statistical methods, usually Student T testing, are useful to contrast maximum and minimum times, and establish that any differences between, for example, real and trough (NADIR) of any rhythm observed were significant statistically.

There are a range of other methods in use,[9,17,18] some especially useful when rhythms are non-sinusoidal or when several rhythms may coexist. Other methods are useful when studying sequential data in one subject both when there is insufficient data for rhythm analysis [Fig 2] or when there is [Fig 3], looking for rhythmicity and then for changes in that rhythmicity [Fig 4].[14-16,19,20]

IV. METHODS

A basic technique of the scientist whose primary interest is biological rhythmicity is the measurement of events at several points, preferable six or more, over many cycles of change. Alternatively one cycle of change can be studied in many subjects and this is the method used in most of the studies described in this article. The results section summarises an abstracted series of reports from the literature that are only a selection of the many that provide the evidence that the immune system is rhythmic.

Both observational and experimental approaches have been used to establish that the immune system in health has variationg that are related to body-time, and that these are predictable and reproducible, both on a 24 hour scale and also on a circumannual or seasonal scale, with other rhythms eg. those with 7-day cycles also having been documented.

Studies fall into two main groups: 1. experimental and 2. field e.g. clinical.

1.   **Experimental studies** that merit serious consideration are done with a full awareness of environmental factors, especially time of light on and light off. In some studies, including some in man, there is a deliberate attempt to reduce many other factors that could cause variance and to control those known to influence rhythmicity. Our experiments in murines were almost all performed in chronobiological isolation chambers that we designed and built for this function. We used timed collections of urine using devices that we designed and made for this purpose to collect samples to study, for example the adrenal rhythm. Manipulation of the lighting in which experimental animals were kept, so that day is 'night' and night is 'day', were possible (and resulted in the circadian variations that we observed in delayed hypersensitivity cell-mediated immune responses reversing, with the time of their maximum transposed by 12 hours). The use of these chambers allowed workers to conduct studies during the "lights off" phase of the animals, but while working "socially acceptable" hours.

2.   **Field studies** have been used for all clinical studies directly concerning immunology that I am aware of, and for all human studies into immune responses, althoush bunkers to study human rhythms are available in a very few centres.

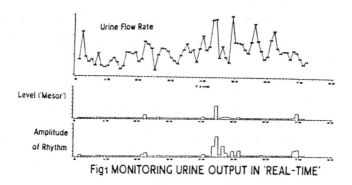

Fig1 MONITORING URINE OUTPUT IN 'REAL-TIME'

Figure 4. Change in amplitude and level of urine flow, collected every 4 hours, is shown in the upper graph, as measured. Analysis using methods of Smith & Gordon[17] and data change in the level (upper histograms) and in the amplitude (lower histograms). Changes resulted from an alteration in treatment with corticosteroid. A change in the developing amplitude of the rhythm, which almost doubles from 0.36 to 0.68, and in the level, which changes from 1.16 to 1.42 was detected with specimen 44, with the change in amplitude already identified from specimen 43. The change in medication was on Day 8 and change was detected with the first specimens of Day 8.

The most usual technique is to take a series of observations in the course of the time-frame of one or more cycles of the suspected rhythms. In many of the reported studies the analysis of data has been retrospective, on data collected for some other purpose but with sufficient density of data to make an analysis for rhythmicity possible. The extent during prospective studies to which there has been an attempt to control other influences, e.g. food, activity, posture, lighting, has varied. In our clinical studies, on the pharmacology of anti-inflammatories and of immuno-modulators the methods mostly have been prospective, using the technique of the double-blind controlled trial, but varying time of an intervention rather than its nature or its dose or intensity. We favoured minimal intervention with life-style and conducted studies in patient's homes. One retrospective survey-based study attempted to link outcome with the time of administration of immuno-modulation. Retrospective information was collected and analysed but there remains uncertainty about its quality because with a lack of awareness that time of administration is important there is doubt about whether the intentions of treating physicians in this regard (if they had any) were followed by patients.

V. RESULTS

Physiological and immunological responses are different at different times. The results in this section are all taken from the published literature and the original publications that provide the evidence that the immune system is rhythmic and that the time of administration of immunomodulating agents can influence their effect, and their toxicity. In this presentation most of the results are presented as example data to illustrate some of the more important conclusions.

Antibody production and the complement cascade are affected by the body's physiological state at the time in the body's rhythms when an immune stimulus is applied. The direct hypersensitivity response in both skin and bronchi show marked circadian variations in magnitude, as does the skin response to histamine. These are not considered in more detail here as they are not the main focus of the paper but are well reviewed in the

Table 1 Early studies of circadian change in cellular immunity.

Circadian variations in human cellular immunity

Cell type	Peak timing Hrs and Min	Circadian Variation (%)
Neutrophil	1932	18
Lymphocytes	0116	34
T_DTH (*in vivo*)	0700	+
T_NK	1115	51
Ts	2156	47
Th	2232	59
B	0043	82

Circadian variations in murine cellular immunity

	Peak timing (Hrs into Light phase of cycle)	Peak timing (Hrs into dark phase of cycle	Circadian Variation (%)
Macrophage function carbon clearance)	8 3/4	–	20
Neutrophils	4	–	72
Lymphocytes	3	–	56
T_DTH (*in vivo*)	–	10 1/2	108
T_NK	–	1 1/2	14

Abstracted from Pownall[21]

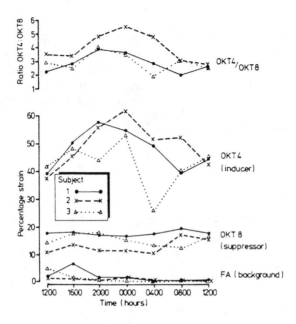

Figure 5. Circadian Variation in OKT4/OKT8 ratio in healthy human males from Knapp.[22]

literature.[3,6]

Circadian variations in the leucocyte, T-cell, B-cell NK-lymphocyte and phagocytic-cell components of the immune response have all been demonstrated to show rhythmic variations as have several T-cell sub-sets[5,22] [Fig 5, Table 1]. There are also seasonal (circumannual) rhythms.[5,16,19]

The total in-vivo cell-mediated immune response when investigated using Oxazalone Sensitivity in the rat, shows a large amplitude circadian rhythm [Fig 1]. This method, noted for its reproducibility and lack of day to day variance (in the hands of some groups), allows quantification of a delayed hypersensitivity response in the rat ear, as reflected by micrometer-measured ear thickness following an oxazalone challenge in sensitised rats. The data in Fig 1 shows that this is only a reproducible response with control of light/dark laboratory conditions and strict standardisation of timing. There is a large change even in the usual working hours of most laboratories, due to the circadian rhythm. The circadian rhythm is light/dark dependent with its cycle reversed when rats are exposed to light at night and darkness by day.[1,2,21,22]

In the healthy human there were also circadian variations demonstrated, established in a study using the tuberculin response in tuberculin sensitive young adults as an example of cell-mediated immune response [Fig 6].[23]

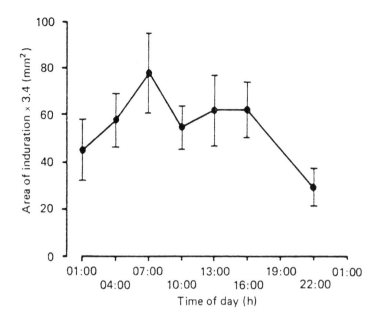

Figure 6. Circadian variation in a cell-mediated response in man.[23]

In the rat we have shown good correlation in time between lymphocyte numbers and delayed hypersensitivity to oxazolone. These variables ghowed an inverse relationship to the corticosterone rhythm. Delayed hypersensitivity and white-cell counts are maximal at the beginning of the light phase when corticosterone levels in the blood are minimal. In man there is less evidence that the circadian pattern of adrenopituitary secretion of cortisol influences T - and B-cell numbers or their activities, for example in lymphocytes during stimulation tests. These very fully documented rhythms of plasma cortisol in man do not show the obvious inverse relationship between levels of adrenal glucocorticoid at certain times with the magnitude of a direct hypersensitivity responses at those times, such as is seen in the rat.[9,21] In studies of lymphocyte numbers at night, during the bursts of adrenal steroid output that preceed waking, we noted only a general correlation between level of cortisol and lymphocyte numbers [Fig 7].

Clinical examples in asthma, rheumatoid arthritis, transplantation and both immediate and delayed-type hypersensitivity reactions in human skin indicate that pathological events involving immune responses do show circadian variations in intensity.

In studies of rheumatoid arthritis, using an experimental design that I consider was well suited to clinical field studies our results[24] demonstrated rhythmicity in symptoms and signs, with the peak of the rhythm in symptoms at the time of the already well described morning time for maximum symptoms [Fig 8], previously attributed to overnight immobility.

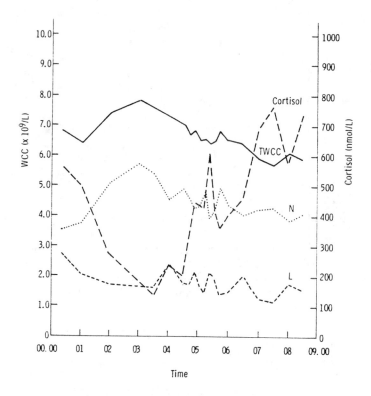

Figure 7 Early morning rising plasma cortisol in a healthy human subject plotted with changes in peripheral white cells.[21]

If these or similar studies were to be repeated I would now request that patients took continuous observations during the "washout" periods between the different timing medication periods studied, as with improved methods for data analysis the period of "washout" can be investigated both for change points in overall trends and for alterations in rhythmicity [Fig 4].[17]

In studies on the response of the airway passages to allergens the peak of a rhythm in immediate sensitivity is seen, from the studies of Reinberg and colleagues in Paris[3] and later workers elsewhere. They demonstrated the relevance of this observation to the nocturnal exacerbations of asthma, which are also in part due to physiological variations in the calibre of airways seen in health and, in an exaggerated pattern, in asthmatics approaching crisis.

In allograft transplantation both animal and human studies have investigated the possibility that rhythms in the immune systems relevant to rejection and tolerance might influence graft survival, or indicate that there is a correct time to give immunomodulating

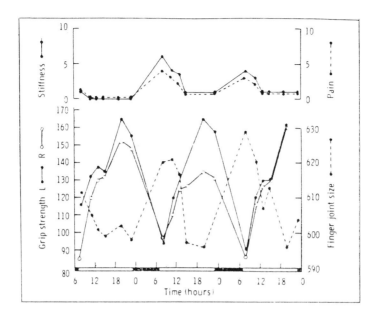

Figure 8. This circadian rhythms of symptoms and signs in patients with Rheumatoid Arthritis is now well documented[24] but it remains uncertain whether the reason for this rhythm is related to rhythms in immune response, in inflammation or to other influences.

treatment. In the renal transplants the numbers of animals investigated in prospective studies have sometimes been inadequate for final conclusions, and in retrospective studies in man the confusing effects of the multiple variables that influence outcome have made conclusions tentative rather than definitive. We suggested that there might be a time of day, or rather of night, when rejection most frequently became manifest. We also confirmed the susgestion of de Vechii, Halberg and others that there is a 7 day periodicity in the occurrence of rejection episodes, with other clinical and experimental results supporting the hypothesis that there may be a seven day cycle in the processes that determine rejection of renal allografts [Fig 9]. There is experimental data after transplantation of cardiac and pancreatic cell allografts that the timing of administration of drugs, in both the circadian and the 7-day rhythms, is an influence on graft survival.[3]

VI. DISCUSSION

It is now certain that the immune system is rhythmic as are the associated processes involved in inflammation. There is now a need to study and explore when these are relevant to a particular question or situation. These rhythms are circadian and seasonal, and there may well also be 7 day rhythms, 12 hour rhythms, 28 day rhythms (especially in the ovulating female) and others of interest or importance.

(A)   Interval between rejection episodes (first 60 days). (All rejections other than solitary events in 48 patients).

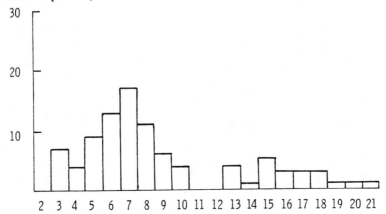

(B)   Distribution of 32 rejection episodes in a 24 h span. Significantly more episodes started between 2300 h and 1100 h than between 1100 h and 2300 h ($\chi^2 = 9.31$; $p < 0.01$)

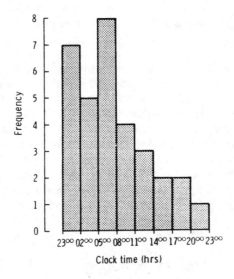

Figure 9.   The timing of rejection episodes after renal allografts in humans suggests: (a) a circadian rhythm; (b) a 7-day rhythm.[2,21]

The most obvious implication of these rhythms is that single time point studies can be misleading. Our present understanding of immunology has been acquired from studies conducted at, or close to, one particular time of day. There are many converts to chronobiology amongst scientists who worked at other times to speed up data collection for publications or other deadlines. They found that systems may behave strangely, with results obtained unlike any before. This is not surprising when an immune response can be easy to detect at 10.00 hours and almost undetectable at 16.00 hours, these two times both being in then working day of most immunologists. Standardisation of the time of day of any investigation will reduce variation, but failure to explore the response at other times may mean that important information is not collected.

Are there any pitfalls in ignoring circadian variation other than to standardise the timing of experiments? Among those that have occurred include the interpretation of observations that there are differences between species in response to the same dose of antigen, as these may not necessarily imply differences in immunological reactivity as they could arise because different animals have different biological rhythms. Rhythms in different species may peak at different times, and this in turn may modify the timins of the peak immune response. A very well documented example is the difference in timing of endogenous corticosteroid rhythms in man and in rodents, related to rats being nocturnal in their activity while man in contrast is diurnally active.

Biological rhythms in animals are influenced by lighting regimens and the effect on the immune response can be dramatic. Rats challenged at 10.00 hours in our laboratories either show delayed hypersensitivity to oxazolone or tolerance with light-dark cycle manipulation [Fig 1]. Rodents are usually maintained on a symmetrical 12h light to 12h dark regimen. this is not the case in the real world for them or for other species. Man is synchronised by an approximate 16 to 18 hour activity to a 6 to 8 hour rest cycle. The symmetrical sinusoidal rhythm of animals in a laboratory with 12:12 light/dark is less obvious in field studies on humans.

The clinical immunologist needs to be alert when shift workers attend allergy or asthma clinics? Those working in behaviourial sciences need to be aware that variables they study may influence rhythmicity and this could influence the immune system indirectly. In some pathological states, notably unipolar depressive illness, there are very well marked disturbances of physiological rhythms and in rhythms of mood, but I am not aware of studies of immunity in such patients, but there might well coexist disturbances in rhythms of immune response.

It is clear from the example of the plasma cortisol level that attention to the timing of procedures is critical to get meaningful results. In tests of immune response the amplitude of the observed rhythms has a similar magnitude, considered as amplitude as a function of mean, to those seen in the level of some hormones. To get better precision from tests of immune function it may be wise to pay as much attention to timing as do endocrinologists.[3,25]

Those investigating immunology should also realise that laboratories that rely on natural daylight are neglecting to standardise an important experimental condition. This is one reason why workers in different geographical locations cannot reproduce results obtained elsewhere. Continuous light in a laboratory can cause very disturbed rhythms, with resulting instability in an animal model.

There is considerable potential to use alterations in lighting regimens or in activity/sleep pattern to help dissect the contributions of different components of immune responses, by observing them during manipulations of lighting regimes, e.g. as experimental subjects move from one schedule of lighting to another, or from one activity cycle, to another. In such experiments the Bayesian "real-time" statistical methods have a useful application.[14-17,19] All components of an immune response may not 'reverse' to the same degree or at the same rate, and theories about the sequence of events might be evaluated during light phase changes and with other chronobiological techniques. In a similar way observations made on nervous system, endocrine system and on behaviour would generate data from which a better understanding of what controls and what influences them could emerge.

There is a potential to increase effectiveness of therapy, or decrease toxicity, by more careful timing of interventions.[6-12] When devising new forms of treatment for any disease or disorder it is interesting and important to know whether there is circadian or other rhythmic variation in the disorder, and in the responses to treatment with the new method or with the alternatives. Test systems might be abandoned or drugs rejected because there is no difference between test and control animals at a single selected time point. It is probable for example that one of the most widely used nonsteroidal anti-inflammatory drugs Indomethacin might have been discarded had the screening tests been done on a diurnally active species, as in rats this medication has almost no anti-inflammatory activity during the dark phase of the 24 hours (and has been shown to have marked time dependant variations in effects in humans). That the timing of an intervention can influence rhythms in systems not normally considered is illustrated by the example of the effect of timing of alternate day dexamethasone treatment on the corneal mitosis rate[26] and by those that showed the effect of the time of BCG inoculations given to protect against tumour growth after implantations into the peritoneum [Fig 10].[26,27]

In clinical practice several situations exist where it is established that taking care over treatment timing is important. There is rather poor compliance with the identified best (or worst) times by patients. This is, often due to ignorance, except in a few situations. With *in-vitro* fertilisation programs, when patients are made well aware of the importance of timing and also of the penalty of incorrect timing (both financial and social) there is great care taken with timing. Often patients are not instructed by their physicians in the best time to take medication, sometimes because physicians are ignorant of this aspect of therapeutics. There has been little effort from most pharmaceutical companies to establish if there is a best or worst time to take most of the medications that are sold and used, and so physicians do not have the information they need.

Rhythmicity appears to be one of the basic properties of the immune system or rhythmicity is a consistent result from a basic rhythmicity in one or other of the other systems that influence the immune system. The complex interaction between the immune system and the rest of the body's cells and physiological organisation pose a challenge for the chronobiologist, for the immunologist and also for those with their interest in any interactions with the Central Nervous System and with the Behavioral Sciences.

Immune responsiveness was changed to apparent tolerance, simply by altering the time of exposure to an antigen.[1,21,22]. At one time of day challenge with antigen results in full expression of the cell-mediated immune response, whereas at another time the same rats, or rats that are similar in every way, show almost no response. Variation in the time of day of challenge does more than 'tinker' with the magnitude of the response, it tips the balance between delayed hypersensitivity and apparent tolerance to the same dose of antigen. Indications are that similar large alterations in other aspects of immune function are also greatly influenced by body-time, and perhaps by alterations in this. If events influencing the brain have an influence on rhythms then it is probable they will influence the immune system.

That rhythmicity should be considered when studying the interactions between brain,

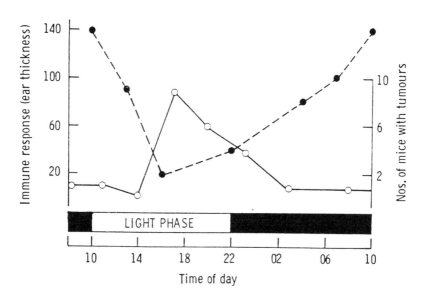

Figure 10. There is a rhythm of immune response in rats. These graphs show results that demonstrate that the time of antigen encounter influences the magnitude of a subsequent cell-mediated immune response (●-●).[13] The results are graphed to contrast with results of studies (also in rats) when it can be seen (○-○) that, in animals injected with tumour cells, but protected against tumour growth by prior immunisation with BCG, that protection was greatest when given at certain times.[26,27] The experiments demonstrated that the time when minimal immune responses were observed was the time when most rats developed tumours, after inoculation with tumour cells. In man, maximal cell-mediated immune responses are observed after early morning challenges. Early morning is the time when rheumatoid patients experience most symptoms.

behaviour and the immune system is emphasised by results that indicate considerable rhythmicity in central nervous system function, and others that demonstrate that the time of therapeutic interventions can influence actions on the nervous system and on behaviour. Some of these data are illustrated, and the topic was reviewed in the publication of Redfern and colleagues.[25] Reports document the effect of sleep deprivation on prolactin rhythms, while other studies suggest that prolactin is an important influence of immuno-regulation. This is only one of several examples where interactions could be anticipated. Seasonal patterns in the presentation of cancer in California might be postulated to be as a result of circumannual changes in the intensity of immune responses.

This review emphasises both the need to consider chronobiology in the course of routine science in all disciplines, and also points out the need for more investigation of whether interactions between the rhythms in different body systems may explain phenomena still unexplained. The review also provides illustrations that indicate the need for more chronbiological awareness in both clinical science and in clinical practice.

The author is grateful to his co-authors in the publications quoted and to many others who have made other contributions working in collaboration, and to those in other independent groups studying chronobiology. Those requiring a more complete bibliography, which is available as computer fileg, should send a disc and return envelope to the author if ASCII files only are required. He will provide references organised as described in reference 18 to those holding a licence to use Paperbase de Luxe. Some chronobiological publications are in publications that may not be easy to access, and the author would be pleased to assist those with difficulties in this regard.

VII. REFERENCES

1. Pownall, R. and Knapp, M.S., Immune responses have rhythms; are they important? *Immunol.Today*, 1, 7, 1980.
2. Knapp, M.S. and Pownall, R., Biological rhythms in cell-mediated immunity. Findings from rats and man and their potential clinical relevance, in *Recent Advances in the Chronobiology of Allergy and Immunology*, Smolensky, M., Reinberg, A. and McGovern, J.P., Eds., Pergamon Press, Oxford, 1979. 323.
3. Levi, F., Reinberg, A. and Canon, C., Clinical immunology and allergy, in *Biological Rhythms in Clincal Practice*, Arendt, J., Minors, D.S. and Waterhouse, J.M., Eds., Butterworths, London, 1989. 99.
4. Levi, F., Canon, C., Blum, J.P., Reinberg, A. and Mathe, G., Large-amplitude circadian rhythm in helper:suppressor ratio of peripheral blood lymphocytes, *Lancet*, ii, 462, 1983.
5. Levi, F., Canon, C., Blum, J.P., Mechkouri, M., Reinberg, A. and Mathe, G., Circadian and/or circahemidian rhythms in nine lymphocyte- related variables from peripheral blood of healthy subjects, *J.Immunol.*, 134, 217, 1985.
6. Smolensky, M.H., Reinberg, A. and McGovern, J.P., *Recent Advances in the Chronobiology of Allergy and Immunology*, Pergamon Press, Oxford, 1979.
7. Kreiger, D.T., *Endocrine Rhythms*, Raven, New York, 1979.
8. Reinberg, A., Smolensky, M. and Labrecque, G., *Annual Review of*

Chronopharmacology; Vol 1, Pergamon, Oxford, 1984.

9.   Arendt, J., Minors, D. and Waterhouse, J.M, *Biological Rhythms in Clinical Practice*, Butterworths, London, 1989.

10.   Hayes, D.K., Pauly, J.E. and Reiter, R.J., *Chronobiology: Its Role in Clinical Medicine, General Biology and Agriculture*, Wiley-Liss, New York, 1990.

11.   Waterfield, J., Growth Factors, *Br.Med.Bull.*, 45, Issue, 1989.

12.   Scheving, L.E., Tsai, T.H. and Scheving, L.A., Circadian dependant responses in DNA synthesis to epidermal growth factor in spleen, bone marrow and lung and in the mitotic index of corneal epithelium, *Prog.Clin.Biol.Res.*, 227a, 1981, 1987.

13.   Pownall, R. and Knapp, M.S., Circadian rhythmicity of delayed hypersensitivity to oxazolone in the rat, *Clin.Sci.Mol.Med.*, 54, 444, 1978.

14.   Knapp, M.S., Computing for clinical chronobiology, for bibliographic compilation and for data storage, graphical representation and statistical analysis, in *Chronobiology: Its Role in Clinical Medicine, General Biology and Agriculture*, Hayes, D.K., Pauley, J.E. and Reiter, R.J., Eds., Wiley-Liss, New York, 1991. 449.

15.   Knapp, M.S., Trimble, I.M., Pownall, R. and Gordon, R., Mathematical and statistical aids to evaluate data from renal patients, *Kid.Int.*, 24, 474, 1983.

16.   Elithorn, A., Psychological testing: The way ahead, in *Current Issues in Clinical Psychology*, Karas, E., Ed., Plenum,Vol 1, London, 1982.

17.   Gordon, K. and Smith, A.F.M., Modelling and monitoring biomedical time series, in *Bayesian Analysis of Time Series and Dynamic Models*, Spall, J., Ed., Dekker, New York, 1988.

18.   De Prins, J., Cornelisson, G. and Malbecq, W., Statistical procedures in chronobiology and chronopharmacology, in *Annual Review of Chronopharmacology, Vol 2*, Pergamon Press, Oxford, 1986. 27.

19.   Smith, A.F.M. and Cook, D.G., Straight lines with a change point: A Beyesian application of some renal transplant data, *Appl.Stats.*, 29, 180, 1980.

20.   Minors, D. and Waterhouse, J.M., Analysis of biological time series, in *Biological Rhythms in Clinical Practice*, Arendt, J., Minors, D. and Waterhouse, J.M., Eds., Butterworths, London, 1989. 27.

21.   Knapp, M.S., Philippens, K.M., Swannell, W., Pownall, R. and Unger, A., Chronobiology and chronotherapeutics, *Br.J.Clin.Prac.*, 38 (Supplement 33), 1, 1984.

22.   Knapp, M.S., Lymphocytes are rhythmic: Is this important, *Br.Med.J.*, 289, 1328, 1984.

23.   Cove-Smith, J.R., Kabler, P., Pownall, R. and Knapp, M.S., Circadian variation in an immune response in man, *Br.Med.J.*, 2, 253, 1978.

24.   Kowanko, I.C., Knapp, M.S., Pownall, R. and Swannell, A.J., Domiciliary self measurement in rheumatoid arthritis and the demonstration of circadian rhythmicity, *Ann Rheum.Dis.*, 42, 453, 1982.

25.   Redfern, P.H., Campbell, I.E., Davies, J.A. and Martin, K.F., *Circadian Rhythms in the Central Nervous System*, McMillan, London, 1984.

26.   Cardosa, S.S., Sowell, J.G. and Goodrum, P.J., Effect of Dexamethasone on Circadian Cell Cycle, in *Chronobiology*, Scheving, , Halberg, and Pauly, , , Eds., Isaho, Tokyo, 1974. 311.

27.   Tsai, T.H., Burns, E.F. and Scheving, L.E., Circadian influence on the immunisation of mice and subsequent challenge with Ehrlich ascites carcinoma, *Chronobiologica*, 6, 187, 1976.

SLEEP DEPRIVATION AND THE IMMUNE RESPONSE TO PATHOGENIC AND NON-PATHOGENIC ANTIGENS

Richard Brown, Gerald Pang[a], Alan J. Husband[a], Maurice G. King, and Diane F. Bull.

Department of Psychology and [a]Faculty of Medicine, The University of Newcastle, NSW. 2308. Australia.

In folklore there exists the belief that one of the best remedies for ailments, especially of an infectious nature, is bed rest and the sleep which accompanies it. This paper reviews the evidence for a role for sleep, in particular slow-wave sleep (SWS), in the progression of infection and the subsequent immune response. Set out below are experimental findings from three areas which lend credence to the proposition that sleep is an integral component of the immune response.

I. EXPERIMENTAL INFECTION

Feelings of sleepiness and lethargy have long been associated with infectious disease states. In the first demonstration of this relationship in a laboratory setting, Krueger and colleagues[1] reported an increase in SWS in rabbits following infection with *Staphylococcus aureus*. The rapid eye movement sleep (REMS) component of sleep was not affected as a result of infection. The most important aspect of this research was the discovery of a significant positive correlation between time spent in SWS and favourable resolution of the infection.

II. MURAMYL PEPTIDES

The brain and body fluids of sleep-deprived animals including man accrue substances which, when extracted and purified, act as potent somnogens. Since the first demonstration of the sleep-inducing properties of cerebrospinal fluid extracted from sleep-deprived dogs,[2] many putative somnogenic substances or "sleep factors" have been proposed. Not the least of which is Factor S which was originally described by Pappenheimer and colleagues in 1967.[3] The successful extraction and purification of Factor S from the brain and body fluids of several sleep deprived mammal species including man[4] led to its identification as a muramyl peptide (MP). This is surprising since MP's are derived from the cell wall of both Gram positive and Gram negative bacterial species[4,5] and cannot be synthesized by mammalian cells.[4] When injected intracerebrally MP's specifically enhance SWS with little effect on REMS[6] and are also among the most powerful immune adjuvants known.[5] MP's are pyrogens as well.[5,6]

As MP's cannot be synthesized by mammalian cells, a putative source of MP's in non-infected mammals is thought to be the gastrointestinal flora, in particular the so-called strictly anaerobic "autochthonous" flora situated close to the intestinal wall.[7-9] This assumption is supported by findings in our laboratory which show a decrease in SWS but not REMS following one week of antibiotic therapy concurrent with an 80% reduction in total anaerobe numbers recoverable from the gut, and a return to normal SWS times one week after cessation of the therapy with a return to normal anaerobe numbers.[10] This phenomenon has also been reported in humans.[11]

Phagocytic cells can digest bacteria and subsequently secrete MP fragments[12] thus producing a ready supply of these molecules within the host. Indeed, recent findings have demonstrated enzyme activity in human serum specific for certain MP structures.[13] Routine absorption of whole bacteria or fragments of bacteria from the gastrointestinal tract and subsequent processing by either the phagocytic or the serum enzyme activity may be the source of the endogenous MP's seen in sleep-deprived mammals.

The potent somnogenic actions of MP's and their apparent increased availability during bacterial infection suggests a mechanism for increased sleep in such disease states. The case of enhanced SWS following administration of viral RNA analogues[14] however is a different matter as there are no MP's associated with viral particles. Another mechanism must be found to explain the sleepiness associated anectdotally with viral infections although it could be argued that in some cases, the increased sleep is due to secondary bacterial infection. This mechanism may be the release of various cytokines and their actions on the brain during the immune response and this possibility is discussed in the next section.

III. CYTOKINES AND SLOW WAVE SLEEP

During the course of an immune response various cytokines are released which target cells both within the immune system and within other systems including the nervous system. For instance receptors for interleukin-l (IL-1) have been reported[15] and brain interleukin-2 acitivity has been observed following brain injury.[16] Recently IL-1 has been identified within neurons of the brain and sympathetic nervous system.[17,18]

Several cytokines have been found to be potent somnogens. IL-1, tumor necrosis factor alpha, and interferon alpha induce large amounts of SWS.[19-21] Recently IL-2 was found to induce sleep when administered specifically into the locus ceruleus the main noradrenergic cell body region in the brain.[22]

It would seem that the initiation of an immune response and hence release of these cytokines in biologically "significant" amounts has the effect of sleep induction. Indeed the adjuvant, fever, and somnogenic effects of MP's are thought to be due to their ability to induce the production and release of IL-1 and possibly other cytokines.[23]

IV. IMMUNE CHANGES DURING SLEEP

Moldofsky and colleagues[24,25] have shown that the immune system is not in a steady state during the sleeping hours. For instance a rapid increase in plasma IL-1 levels is associated with the onset of SWS with a similar increase in IL-2 occuring shortly after this event. Increases in mitogen response and a dramatic fall natural killer cell activity were also seen and may be the result of the IL-1 and IL-2 availability during sleep. The enhanced SWS in infected organisms has yet to be examined in terms of sleep-related changes in immune function. Such an undertaking would be highly informative.

V. SLEEP DEPRIVATION AND IMMUNITY

Table 1 summarises the effects of sleep loss in the animal and human studies mentioned below.

The veracity of a sleep-immunity relationship may be tested under conditions where the immune-related function(s) of sleep is subtracted from the ongoing immune response. The difference in outcome between sleep-deprived subjects and controls may be reasonably ascribed to the missing input of sleep to the response. There is a caveat however and this is associated with "stress" of both psychological and physiological nature as a result of loss of sleep. While this stress may not be great in humans possessing full knowledge of the situation and indeed who are motivated to remain awake, the case of the laboratory animal is quite different. Therefore any discussion of the effects of sleep loss on immunity must be considered in relation to any possible stress effects due to sleep loss and any interaction between this stressor and the "genuine" effects of sleep loss.

Most studies of sleep loss and immunity have shown what can only be described as minor perturbations in immune function. For instance, fluctuations in white blood cell numbers have been observed in humans and animals following several days sleep loss[26-28] and Palmblad and colleagues[29] have reported that a combination of battle stress and total sleep loss for three days resulted in depressed phagocytic activity and enhanced interferon secretion which persisted several days efter the sleep loss vigil. The clinical relevance of such changes is not known.

One of the problems with the interpretation of most of the findings in Table 1. is that these experiments were done on animals and humans who were not undergoing any immune response coincident with sleep loss. In effect the immune measures presented above are reflections of in vitro rather than in vivo immune activity as has been previously pointed out by Benca et al.[30] Many of these studies examined individuals who were not undergoing an immune response, particularly a response to a pathogen.

In order to gain a clearer understanding of the effect of sleep loss on immunity we tested animals and humans who were deliberately infected with either virulent or innocuous antigens immediately prior to extended periods of wakefullness. With the immune system activated in this manner it could be expected that any effects of sleep loss would be evidentin the response of the animal in terms of its ability to deal with the antigen challenge compared to challenged but sleeping controls.

We have shown that rats challenged with sheep red blood cells at the commencement of 8 hours sleep deprivation displayed reduced antibody titres to SRBC three days post-

Table 1. Effects of Sleep Deprivation on the Immune System

Animal Studies:

Manaceine[26] : 4-5 days in puppies ⇒ Lowered white blood cell count

Kleitman[16] : 2-7 days in puppies ⇒ No change in white blood cell count

Solomon[32] : REM deprivation 2 days pre/post challenge in rats ⇒ Decreased primary but not secondary response to sheep erythrocytes

Casey *et al*[33] : REM deprivation 3 days in mice ⇒ Increased uptake of sheep erythrocytes in peritoneal macrophages; Decreased uptake in spleen and liver

Rechtschaffen *et al*[34] : 30 days in rats ⇒ Decreased spleen size

Benca *et al*[30] : Up to 30 days in rats ⇒ No change in splenocyte proliferation

Brown *et al*[31] : 8 hours immediately post-challenge in rats ⇒ Decreased antibody formation to sheep erythrocytes reversible by pretreatment with IL-1 beta or MDP

Brown *et al*[35] : 7 hours immediately post-challenge in mice ⇒ Corruption of immunity to influenzae virus and depleted IgA in lung

---

Human Studies:

Kuhn *et al*[36] : 4 days ⇒ Increased white blood cell count

Palmblad *et al*[28] : 3 days plus battle simulation ⇒ Decreased phagocytosis of viral particles and increased interferon secretion persisting post-vigil

Palmblad *et al*[29] : 3 days ⇒ Decreased granulocyte and lymphocyte proliferation

Moldofsky *et al*[25] : 40 hours ⇒ Increased nocturnal release of IL-1 and IL-2; Delayed nocturnal rise in response to pokeweed mitogen; Depressed natural killer cell activity persisting beyond vigil

Brown *et al* (in preparation) : 24 hours commencing at antigen administration ⇒ Enhanced PWM-induced IgM secretion in blood culture and salivary IgA and IgG against 5. typhi on day 7; Enhanced serum IgA on Day 14 post secondary challenge and enhanced IgA secretion in blood culture on days 7-14 post secondary challenge.

---

deprivation.[31] An important finding of this study was the ability of both IL-1 and MDP to prevent this suppression when given in conjuction with SRBC challenge. Interestingly we also found that doses of both IL-1 and MDP at concentrations which are immunosuppressive in non-deprived rats, also prevented the sleep deprivation-induced suppression of anti-SRBC antibody titres. We are currently unable to explain this effect.

To examine the effect of sleep loss on the progression of a disease state we employed an influenza model in Swiss albino mice.[35] These mice were challenged intranasally with a dose of virulent influenza virus at the commencement of 7 hours sleep deprivation.

Analysis at 3 days post deprivation revealed an average $10^{2.93}$ viral particles per ml of lung homogenate in sleep deprived mice. This was in stark contrast to normal mice who showed no viral particles whatsoever in lung homogenates. This disease state was probably due to the significantly reduced IgA titres observed in lungs of sleep deprived mice. The most startling aspect of this study was the fact that all mice had been immunized previously against the influenza virus.

In a recent experiment with humans we have examined the effects of twenty four hours sleep deprivation on the kinetics of mucosal antibody production following oral challenge with a *Salmonella typhi* mutant (Typh-Vax vaccine). Subjects were given one Typh Vax capsule containing 109 live *S. typhi* mutant on the morning of the sleep deprivation night. The aim was to separate antigen challenge from the next sleep period by at least 24 hours. Results showed a surge of anti *S. typhi* IgA and IgG in saliva 7 days after challenge in the sleep deprived group as well as enhanced mitogen-driven secretion of IgM at this time.

When challenged with a second Typh-Vax dose 8 weeks later there were significant increases in serum IgA 14 days post-challenge and in IgA secretion in blood cultures 7-14 days post-challenge.

The alterations in antibody production seen in this study suggest that the host response to a potentially pathogenic organism like *S. tyhpi* is markedly altered following sleep loss at a critical period, namely at initial challenge. At present it is not known if these changes are clinically relevant. However if the influenza model in the mouse[35] is any indication, then such fluctuations of immune response should be considered to be of great importance when it comes to the "bottom line" namely of protection against disease.

VI. CONCLUSIONS

From the experimental evidence presented above conclusions may be drawn regarding the involvement of SWS and the function of the immune system. Firstly, there appears to be a potent somnogenic signal carried to the brain via several key cytokines. While this effect may well be dismissed as artefact if only one substance produced this effect on the brain, the growing list of substances, both endogenous and of bacterial and viral origin which induce SWS suggests otherwise. Secondly, the positive relationship between recovery from a pathogenic challenge and the amount of time the host spends in SWS is suggestive of a facilitatory role for SWS in the immune response. Thirdly the finding that sleep loss, particularly in subjects challenged with virulent antigen, interferes with the immune response is perhaps the most convincing evidence to date that sleep, most likely SWS, is an important factor contributing to a competent immune response.

VII. REFERENCES

1. Toth, L. and Krueger, J.M., Staphylococcus aureus alters sleep patterns in rabbits, *Infect.Immun.*, 56, 1785, 1988.

2. Legendre, R. and Pieron, H., Le probleme des facteurs sommiel. Resultants d'injections vasculaires et intracerebrales de liquides insomniques, *CR Soc.Biol.*, 68, 1077, 1910.

3. Pappenheimer, J.R., Miller, T.B. and Goodrich, C.A., Sleep-promoting effects of cerebrospinal fluid from sleep- deprived goats, *Proc.Natl.Acad.Sci.USA*, 58, 513, 1967.

4. Pappenheimer, J.R., Induction of sleep by muramyl peptides, *J.Physiol.*, 336, 1, 1983.

5. Chedid, L., Synthetic muramyl peptides; Their origin, present status, and future prospects, *Fed.Proc.*, 45, 2545, 1991.

6. Krueger, J.M., Toth, L.A., Cady, A.B., Johannsen, L. and Obal, F., Immunomodulation and sleep, in *Sleep Peptides: Basic and Clinical Applications*, Inoue, S. and Schneider-Helmert, D., Eds., Japan Science Society Press, Tokyo, 1988.

7. Foo, M.C. and Lee, A., Immunological responses of mice to members of the autochthonous intestinal microflora, *Infect.Immun.*, 6, 525, 1972.

8. Foo, M.C., Lee, A. and Cooper, G.N., Natural antibodies and the intestinal flora of rodents, *Aust.J.Exp.Biol.Med.Sci.*, 52, 321, 1974.

9. Brown, R., Price, R.J., King, M.G. and Husband, A.J., Autochthonous intestinal bacteria and coprophagy: a possible contribution to the ontogeny and rhythmicity of slow wave sleep, *Med.Hypotheses*, 26, 171, 1991.

10. Brown, R., Price, R.J., King, M.G. and Husband, A.J., Are antibiotic effects on sleep behavior in the rat due to modulation of gut bacteria? *Physiol.Behav.*, 48, 561, 1990.

11. Rhee, Y-H. and Kim, H-L., The correlation between sleeping-time and numerical change of intestinal normal flora in psychiatric insomnia patients, *Bull.Naztl.Sci.Chungbuk Natl.Univ.*, 1, 159, 1987.

12. Vermeulen, M.W. and Gray, G.R., Processing of Bacillus Subtilis peptidoglycan by a mouse macrophage cell line, *Infect.Immun.*, 46, 476, 1984.

13. Vanderwinkel, E., De Vlieghere, M., De Pauw, P., Cattalini, N., Ledoux, V., Gigot, D. and Ten Have, J.P., Purification and characterization of N-acetylmuramoyl-L-alanine amidase from human serum, *Biochim.Biophys.Acta*, 1039, 331, 1990.

14. Endersly, J., Ahokas, R.A., Majde, J.A., Blatteis, C.M. and Krueger, J.M., Enhancement of slow-wave sleep by polyriboinosinic: polyribocytidylic acid, *Fed.Proc.*, 46, 1128, 1987.

15. Pert, C.B., Ruff, M.R., Weber, R.J. and Herkenham, M., Neuropeptides and their receptors: A psychosomatic network, *J.Immunol.*, 135, 820s, 1985.

16. Nieto-Sampedro, M. and Chandy, K.G., Interleukin-2-like activity in injured rat brain, *Neurochem.Res.*, 12, 723, 1987.

17. Breder, C.D., Dinarello, C.A. and Saper, C.B., Interleukin-1 immunoreactive innervation of the human hypothalamus, *Science*, 240, 321, 1988.

18. Schultzberg, M., Svenson, S.B., Unden, A. and Bartfai, T., Interleukin-1 like immunoreactivity in peripheral tissues, *J.Neurosci.Res.*, 18, 184, 1987.

19. Krueger, J.M., Walter, J., Dinarello, C.A., Wolff, S.M. and Chedid, L., Sleep-promoting effects of endogenous pyrogen (interleukin-1), *Am.J.Physiol.*, 246, R994, 1984.

20. Shoham, S., Davenne, D., Cady, A.B., Dinarello, C.A. and Krueger, J.M., Recombinant tumor necrosis factor and interleukin-1 enhance slow- wave sleep in rabbits, *Am.J.Physiol.*, 253, R142, 1987.

21. Krueger, J.M., Shoham, S., Davenne, D., Walter, J. and Kubillus, S., Interferon alpha-2 enhances slow-wave sleep in rabbits, *Int.J.Immunopharmacol.*, 9, 23, 1987.

22. Nistico, G. and de Sarro, G., Locus ceruleus: site of soporific effects of interleukin-2 in rats, *Prog.Neuroendocrinimmunol.*, 3, 43, 1190.

23. Dinarello, C.A. and Krueger, J.M., Induction of interleukin-1 by synthetic and naturally occuring muramyl peptides, *Fed.Proc.*, 45, 2545, 1986.

24. Moldofsky, H., Lue, F.A., Eisen, J., Keystone, E. and Gorczynski, R.M., The relationship of interleukin-1 and immune functions to sleep in humans, *Psychosom.Med.*, 48, 309, 1986.

25. Moldofsky, H., Lue, F.A., Davidson, J.R. and Gorczynski, R.M., Effects of sleep deprivation on human immune functions, *FASEB J.*, 1972, 1989.

26. Manaceine, *Arch.Ital.de Biol.*, 21, 322, 1894.

27. Kleitman, N., The effects of prolonged sleeplessness on man, *Am.J.Physiol.*, 66, 67, 1923.

28. Palmblad, J., Cantell, K., Strander, H., Froberg, J., Karlsson, C.G., Levi, L., Granstom, M. and Unger, P., Stressor exposure and immunological response in man: Interferon- producing capacity and phagocytosis, *J.Psychosom.Res.*, 20, 193, 1976.

29. Palmblad, J., Petrini, B., Wasserman, J. and Akerstedt, T., Lymphocyte and granulocyte reactions during sleep deprivation, *Psychosom.Res.*, 41, 273, 1979.

30. Benca, R.M., Kushida, C.A., Everson, C.A., Bergmann, B.M. and Rechtschaffen, A., Sleep deprivation in the rat: VI. Immune function, *Sleep*, 12, 47, 1989.

31. Brown, R., Price, R.J., King, M.G. and Husband, A.J., Interleukin-1 and muramyl dipeptide can prevent decreased antibody response associated with sleep deprivation, *Brain Behav.Immun.*, 3, 320, 1989.

32. Solomon, G.F., Stress and antibody response in rats, *Int.Archs Allergy*, 35, 97, 1969.

33. Casey, F.B., Eisenberg, J., Peterson, D. and Pieper, D., Altered antigen uptake and distribution due to exposure to extreme environmental temperatures and sleep deprivation, *J.Reticuloendothel.Soc.*, 15, 87, 1974.

34. Rechtschaffen, A., Gilliland, M.A., Bergmann, S.M. and Winter, J.B., Physiological correlates of prolonged sleep deprivation in rats, *Science*, 221, 182, 1983.

35. Brown, R., Pang, G., Husband, A.J. and King, M.G., Suppression of immunity to influenza virus infection in the respiratory tract following sleep disturbance, *Reg.Immunol.*, 2, 321, 1989.

36. Kuhn, E., Brodan, V., Brodanova, M. and Rysanek, K., Metabolic reflection of sleep deprivation, *Activ.Nerv.Super.*, 11, 165, 1969.

IV. Life Events, Exercise and Immunity

BEREAVEMENT AND LONG TERM MORBIDITY: AN AUSTRALIAN PROJECT

Roger Bartrop, Lina Forcier, Michael Jones[a], Rosie Kubb, Elizabeth Luckhurst[b] and Ronald Penny[b].

The Department of Academic Psychiatry, University of Sydney at the Royal North Shore Hospital, Sydney, Australia, [a]Health Information Systems Department, Royal North Shore Hospital, Sydney, Australia, and [b]Centre for Immunology, St Vincents Hospital, Sydney, Australia.[*]

I. ABSTRACT

Spouse-bereaved subjects who had participated in earlier bereavement studies volunteered to allow investigation of their health up to eleven years after the death of their spouse. Re-enrolled controls were also studied over a similar period. Morbidity was measured in three ways: self-reports from the subjects, data obtained from medical records, and morbidity data common to both sources (confirmed data). The findings showed that the bereaved had an elevation in morbidity rate over non-bereaved,which was both substantial and statistically significant. Diseases of the circulatory system were significantly more common in the bereaved, as were psychiatric disorders in all data sources. Furthermore, bereaved had more respiratory and musculo-skeletal system illnesses according to the self-report source. Overall, more bereaved than controls suffered at least one illness, and had illnesses of a longer duration. Bereaved with a high level of morbidity in the two years following bereavement also had more illnesses in later years.

II. INTRODUCTION

Bereavement is a common life event which demands research attention. In 1986, 7% of the Australian population were widowed. When this figure is examined by age, 10% of Australians between the ages of 55 to 64, and 35% of those 65 years of age and over were spouse bereaved.[1] In the future, with an ageing population, the proportion of spouses coping with an ill partner and subsequent bereavement is expected to increase.

Short-term morbidity after bereavement has been researched at intervals since the 1950's.[2-5] These reports have generally included non-specific complaints (vegetative symptoms, dysphoric mood and pain syndromes). Other symptoms (yearning, restless behaviour and perceptual phenomena) were more likely to be identified as uniquely grief-related. Only rarely have attempts been made to categorise short and long term concomitants of such distress as

---

[*] Additional statistical assistance was provided by Dr. Michael Adena, Instat Australia, Canberra, Australia.

entities identifiable within an international coding system.

From 1975 until 1977 inclusive, the short-term effects of bereavement were examined in a bereavement project in Sydney, Australia.[6-8] Immunological function in a matched cohort of 26 bereaved subjects demonstrated significant depression of T cell responsiveness to mitogenic stimulation in the bereaved compared to their controls. Since these studies, other workers have demonstrated changes in immunological function in bereaved spouses.[9-11]

The aim of the present study was to investigate retrospectively the health consequences of bereavement for up to 11 years following their loss in the 1975-1977 subjects mentioned above.

III. METHOD

SUBJECTS

For this current follow-up study, the 178 potential subjects who had taken part in the 1975-77 studies were to be asked for information regarding their health (physical and psychiatric morbidity) in a retrospective survey. The time period covered the years from 1975, 1976 or 1977 until December 1985, giving a potential follow-up time of 11 years. Of these individuals, one was discovered to have feigned bereavement. Accordingly, this subject and his control were excluded. Therefore the potential study population was 176 subjects comprising 88 bereaved and 88 controls. Only two subjects could not be found: one bereaved and one control. Of the 174 remaining subjects, 11 had died (five bereaved and six controls). Their families gave consent for the authors to obtain their death certificates. Of the remaining 163 subjects, 11 people declined to be re-enrolled. A total of 152 surviving subjects (72 bereaved and 80 controls) therefore agreed to be re-enrolled in the follow-up morbidity study.

The subjects who declined (10 bereaved spouses and one non-bereaved control) were prepared to give reasons for their refusal and to provide some details about their health. All 10 bereaved declined to participate because they did not wish to relive the experience. Two of them had lost another nuclear family member within the previous six months. Six of them had had a recent depressive illness and, of these six, two also had a substance abuse problem; three of the remaining four bereaved who did not suffer a recent depressive illness had a substance abuse problem. The control who declined did so because of the imminent death of a close family member. She maintained that she had been healthy.

DATA COLLECTION

With living subjects, a record of morbidity over the follow-up period was established twice: once in an interview with the subject ('self-report' data), using a version of the health history approach used by the Australian Veterans' Health Studies[12] and once using records obtained from their general practitioners, and/or specialists, and/or hospital record(s) as appropriate ('record' data). Further, morbidity data which were found in both these sources (matched on both types of disease and time of occurrence) were called 'confirmed' morbidity data. All data were collected by medically qualified persons.

A questionnaire was also administered to each subject to obtain sociodemographic variables and other possible health confounding variables. The details of methods of subject recruitment, data collected on surviving subjects, death certificate data and methods of statistical analysis will be published.[13]

STATISTICAL ANALYSIS

For the data analysis, morbidity level was assessed by using a derived illness score. Calculating morbidity rates as the number of illnesses incurred during the time of the study ignores the duration of the illness(es) and hence neglects an entire dimension to morbidity. For this reason an illness score for each subject was derived; this illness-score was calculated by counting for each disease the number of years in which the disease occurred, then adding counts for all diseases for that subject.

Subjects were asked to recall only the year in which illnesses occurred as this was the smallest unit of time which subjects could confidently recall as the beginning and end to an illness. For example, an illness commencing in January 1976 and terminating in June 1976 added one to the illness-score of that subject while an illness commencing in January 1978 and terminating in June 1979 added another two to that subject's illness-score.

It should be stressed again that in some Tables (Tables 3, 4, 9) presented in this paper the number of illnesses which have occurred is listed rather than the illness-score. When this occurs, it may appear that there is little difference between bereaved and non-bereaved since the difference between the number of diseases in each group is small. However it should be remembered that the number of diseases, on its own, is not an appropriate measure for comparing morbidity between bereaved and non-bereaved. It does not take into account the differing number of subjects contributing illnesses or the differing length of follow-up in each group.

Two types of data analyses were conducted. The first compared subject characteristics, such as age and sex distributions, between the bereaved and control groups. The second compared morbidity rates between the two groups, after controlling for potentially confounding factors.

The former analyses were conducted, in the case of continuous variables such as age, by unpaired t-tests[14] Wilcoxin Rank Sum tests[15] if the data being analysed were not consistent with a normal distribution. Table 8 reports medians and interquartile ranges. The median represents the 50th percentile of the distribution while the interquartile range provides the 25th and 75th percentiles. In the case of discrete factors, such as sex or occupation, Pearson chi-square tests were employed.[15] Unpaired analyses were used since the natural loss of follow-up meant that, of the subjects remaining, there were only 67 complete pairs out of the 89 original pairs of subjects.

Morbidity rates were analysed using log-linear regression.[16] The parameter estimates of the model can be transformed into relative morbidity rates, comparing the bereaved to the control group, while the standard error of the estimate enables confidence intervals to be constructed and hypothesis tests to be conducted. This methodology also allows for i) unequal periods at risk which is made-up of unequal numbers of subjects and individual follow-up times and ii) adjustments to be made to the comparison of bereaved and control morbidity rates for potentially confounding factors, ie. covariance analysis.

Descriptive statistics, Pearson chi-square tests, t-tests, and Mann-Whitney tests were conducted using BMDP[17] and SPIDA.[18] Log linear regression was conducted using GLIM.[19]

IV. RESULTS

SOCIODEMOGRAPHIC, LIFE-STYLE DATA AND OTHER VARIABLES IN THE STUDY POPULATION

In the 1975 to 1977 studies, bereaved had been matched to non-bereaved for some sociodemographic characteristics. However, with unequal loss to follow-up between bereaved and controls, all characteristics had to be examined in this study (Table 1): the 72 live bereaved were compared with the 80 live controls.

Table 1. Variables examined in the analysis

SUBJECT RELATED
   Sex *
   Age *
   Marital Status *
   Body Mass Index (BMI) *
   Weight changes during the follow-up period
   Chronic medication regimen (presence or absence) *
   Smoking status *
   Alcohol consumption *
   Occupation (subject) *
   Occupation (spouse) *
   Subject's judgement of his/her financial status *
   Net weekly income *

STUDY DESIGN RELATED
   Subsequent bereavement during the follow-up period
   Year of subject enrolment
   Method of interview (subject) *
   Method of interview (doctor) *
   Interviewer variability *

* as measured at the time of interview in the follow-up study

MORBIDITY FOLLOW-UP TO DECEMBER 1985 - UNADJUSTED

Only five bereaved and six control subjects had died. The small number of deaths precluded a formal analysis of mortality rates. Morbidity results presented in this part pertain to both physical and psychiatric morbidity. The average follow-up period for study subjects was 10 years for self-report morbidity data and 8.4 years for the record and confirmed morbidity sources. All sources of morbidity data indicated a statistically significant elevation of bereaved morbidity rates over that of controls (Table 2). Using the results of Table 2, according to the record source, bereaved subjects each accrued on average the equivalent of 18.9 illness-score over the eleven year maximum possible follow-up compared with 14.8 illness-score for controls; bereaved subject therefore suffered the equivalent of 4.1 illness-score more than the non-bereaved.

Three bereaved subjects and two controls became spouse bereaved again since they enrolled in the 1975 to 1977 studies. However, exclusion of these subjects did not greatly change the results (Table 2). Accordingly, these subjects were retained in subsequent analyses.

MORBIDITY DATA SOURCES: SELF-REPORT COMPARED WITH RECORD MORBIDITY SOURCE

As noted earlier, both subjects' recollection of their illness history and data from their medical practitioner(s) records were sought. Table 3 shows that, of the 1365 illnesses reported, only 22% were reported by both sources (and therefore made up the confirmed morbidity data source). Approximately 55% of illnesses reported by subjects were not found in the medical records (record source), and approximately 70% of illnesses present in medical records were not mentioned by subjects (Table 3).

The bereaved made statistically significantly more visits to their general practitioners than the nonbereaved (KW = 9.79, p < 0.001). On average for the 11 years of follow-up, bereaved subjects had 51 visits compared with an average of 35 for the non-bereaved.

MORBIDITY FOLLOW-UP TO DECEMBER 1985 - ADJUSTED

Differences were found between bereaved and non-bereaved subjects for their distribution of occupational, financial and medication-related variables. Analyses which adjusted for the different distributions of these variables were performed, as well as analyses adjusting for an the other variables as shown in Table 1.

With the morbidity data obtained from subject reports (self-report source), none of the factors listed in Table 1 explained the effect of bereavement. That is, after controlling for these factors, individually, the difference between the bereaved and the controls was still significant (the adjusted relative morbidity rate ranged from 1.19 to 1.44 and the largest p-value was 0.0006. Results were similar with the morbidity data obtained from record reports. After controlling for each factor listed in Table 1, individually, the adjusted relative morbidity rate ranged from 1.11 to 1.33 and the largest p- value was 0.01.

With confirmed morbidity data, only three factors had a significant effect on the relative morbidity rate. After controlling for the use of chronic medications, the relative morbidity rate (RMR) was 1.04 (with 95% confidence intervals of 0.93 to 1.17 and a p-value of 0.5). After controlling for marital status the RMR was 1.17 (with 95% confidence

Table 2. Summary of relative morbidity rates for bereaved compared with non-bereaved at full follow-up time (unadjusted data).

Morbidity Data Source	Illness-Score[4] Bereaved	Non-Bereaved	Relative Morbidity Rate	95% Conf. Interval	p-value
All Subjects					
Self-Report[1]	1439	1133	1.4	1.3, 1.5	<0.0001
Record[2]	1359	1181	1.3	1.2, 1.4	<0.0001
Confirmed[3]	620	542	1.3	1.1, 1.4	<0.0001
Excluding subjects (bereaved and controls) who had a spouse bereavement since their 1975 - 1977 enrolment					
Self-Report[1]	1274	963	1.4	1.3, 1.5	<0.0001
Record[2]	1220	965	1.4	1.3, 1.5	<0.0001
Confirmed[3]	561	435	1.4	1.2, 1.6	<0.0001

1 - as obtained from study subject
2 - as obtained from general practitioner(s), specialist(s) or hospital records
3 - as found in both the self-report and record sources
4 - results are based on illness-score, not only the number of illnesses (see statistical analysis section for the definition of illness score).

Table 3. Concordance between self-report and record sources of morbidity

	DATA FOUND IN				
Group	Self-report source only	Record source only	Both sources[1]	unique Illnesses	Number of Subjects
Bereaved	197	342	154	693	72
(%)	28	49	22	100	
Controls	176	350	146	672	80
(%)	26	52	22	100	

1 - this is the "confirmed source" which is derived from morbidity data found in both the self-report and record sources

Table 4. Illness incidence in the bereaved: Observed and expected

Years after Enrolled	Number of **New** Illnesses					
	Self-report Source		Record Source		Confirmed Source	
	Obs	Exp[1]	Obs	Exp[1]	Obs	Exp[1]
0	85	48	76	70	37	27
1	24	19	40	29	9	7
2	21	11	30	30	9	5
3	23	27	33	38	12	16
4	21	38	36	36	11	18
5	29	37	40	56	11	18
6	31	29	47	53	13	13
7	45	40	69	50	23	17
8	22	47	64	54	13	17
9	35	46	49	65	12	15
10	15	4	12	15	4	1
Total	351	351	496	496	154	154
Chi-Square (10 df)	34.9		11.9		10.3	
	$p < 0.0001$		$p = 0.3$		$p = 0.5$	

1 - Number of illnesses expected to originate each year after bereavement if the rate of occurrence of new illnesses in the bereaved group is the same as that in the control group.

intervals of 0.98 to 1.40, $p = 0.07$). After controlling for occupation of the spouse the RMR was 1.14 (with 95% confidence intervals of 1.00 to 1.29, $p = 0.05$). It should be noted, however, that medication use could be an outcome variable rather than a true confounder.

In brief, of all the variables examined few had an impact on the relative morbidity rates and, at that, only in one morbidity data source (ie. confirmed). Therefore it is concluded that the estimated difference in morbidity between the bereaved and controls cannot simply be ascribed to confounding by demographic/methodological factors.

Table 5. ICD-9 group and relative morbidity rate (RMR) for the ICD-9 groups in which the morbidity among the bereaved was shown to be elevated or depressed to a statistically significant extent at 1 year, 2 years or full follow-up time (**self-report sources of morbidity data only**)

			Time After Bereavement			
		1 year		2 years		FFT[3]
ICD-9 Group[1]	RMR[2]	95% Confidence Interval	RMR[2]	95% Confidence Interval	RMR[2]	95% Confidence Interval
Neoplasms	-	-, -	-	-, -	3.3[+]	1.8, 6.2
Mental	3.9[+]	1.9, 8.0	4.4[+]	2.4, 8.1	2.7[+]	2.1, 3.5
Neurological	0.4	0.2, 1.2	0.5	0.2, 1.0	0.6'	0.5, 0.9
Circulatory	4.4[+]	2.1, 9.4	4.2[+]	2.3, 7.4	2.0[+]	1.6, 2.5
Respiratory	1.6[*]	1.0, 2.7	1.6'	1.1, 2.4	1.4[+]	1.2, 1.7
Endocrine	2.8	0.5, 14.8	3.0	0.8, 11.4	1.9'	1.2, 3.0
Digestive	1.9	0.8, 4.3	1.7	0.9, 3.2	1.5'	1.1, 1.9
Skin	0.5	0.2, 1.2	0.4[*]	0.2, 0.9	0.5[+]	0.4, 0.7
Injury	5.6	0.6, 48.6	8.9[*]	1.1, 73.6	1.7[*]	1.0, 2.8
Total	1.9[+]	1.5, 2.4	1.9[+]	1.6, 2.3	1.4[+]	1.3, 1.5

1 - grouped according to the 17 major categories of the ICD-9 code (roman numerals)
2 - RMR: relative morbidity rate based on accumulated disease to that point in time
3 - FFT: full follow-up time
* = $p < 0.05$; ' = $p < 0.01$; + = $p < 0.001$; - = no result possible

MORBIDITY RATES OVER TIME

An examination of the cumulative data at yearly intervals after bereavement shows that at all times, the elevation among bereaved was statistically significant. In some cases, the relative morbidity rates decrease between two years and full follow-up time (Tables 5-7) but the majority remain substantial and statistically significant.

When a yearly examination of cumulative relative morbidity rates is performed for the full follow-up time in this project, it is seen that, irrespective of the morbidity source, in each year studied, the higher morbidity rate of bereaved when compared with controls reached statistical significance.

Table 6. ICD-9 group and relative morbidity rate (RMR) for the ICD-9 groups in which the morbidity among the bereaved was shown to be elevated or depressed to a statistically significant extent at 1 year, 2 years or full follow-up time (**record report source of morbidity data only**)

	Time After Bereavement					
	1 year		2 years		FFT[3]	
ICD-9 Group[1]	RMR[2]	95% Confidence Interval	RMR[2]	95% Confidence Interval	RMR[2]	95% Confidence Interval
Mental	2.1*	1.1, 3.8	2.0*	1.2, 3.3	2.1+	1.7, 2.7
Circulatory	3.6*	1.8, 7.3	3.5+	2.0, 6.0	2.0+	1.6, 2.4
Endocrine	1.2	0.3, 4.8	1.2	0.4, 3.4	1.5	1.0, 2.2
Total	1.4ꞌ	1.1, 1.7	1.3+	1.1, 1.6	1.3+	1.2, 1.4

1 - grouped according to the 17 major categories of the ICD-9 code (roman numerals)
2 - RMR: relative morbidity rate based on accumulated disease to that point in time
3 - FFT: full follow-up time
* = $p < 0.05$; ꞌ = $p < 0.01$; + = $p < 0.001$; - = no result possible

Table 7. ICD-9 group and relative morbidity rate (RMR) for the ICD-9 groups in which the morbidity among the bereaved was shown to be elevated or depressed to a statistically significant extent at 1 year, 2 years or full follow-up time (**confirmed report source of morbidity data only**)

	Time After Bereavement					
	1 year		2 years		FFT[3]	
ICD-9 Group[1]	RMR[2]	95% Confidence Interval	RMR[2]	95% Confidence Interval	RMR[2]	95% Confidence Interval
Mental	3.8*	1.2, 12.0	3.7ꞌ	1.5, 9.5	2.7+	1.8, 4.1
Circulatory	2.9*	1.3, 6.3	2.9ꞌ	1.6, 5.5	1.7+	1.4, 2.2
Endocrine	1.2	0.2, 8.7	1.2	0.2, 6.0	2.6ꞌ	1.3, 5.0
Injury	-	-, -	_	-, -	2.4*	1.1, 5.2
Total	1.6ꞌ	1.1, 2.3	1.6+	1.2, 2.1	1.3+	1.1, 1.4

1 - grouped according to the 17 major categories of the ICD-9 code (roman numerals)
2 - RMR: relative morbidity rate based on accumulated disease to that point in time
3 - FFT: full follow-up time
* = $p < 0.05$; ꞌ = $p < 0.01$; + = $p < 0.001$; - = no result possible

WHEN DOES THE INCREASED MORBIDITY OCCUR? YEARLY OBSERVATIONS ON ILLNESS INCIDENCE

The temporal distribution of new illness occurrence among bereaved subjects is compared to that of controls. We take the temporal distribution of new control illnesses as being 'normal' and judge the 'normality' of bereaved relative to this standard. For each year following bereavement we compute the number of new illnesses we expect in the bereaved if they had experienced the same proportion of their new illnesses in that year as the controls. Thus in Table 4 we have, for each data source, the number of new illnesses the bereaved actually experienced each year (observed) and the number they would have experienced if they had the same temporal distribution of new illnesses as the controls (expected). An increase in new illnesses was most evident in the first few years following bereavement (Table 4).

TYPE OF MORBIDITY: ICD-9 CATEGORIES

The morbidity data were coded using the ICD-9 coding system[20] and were grouped under the 17 broad categories of that system. Morbidity coded in this fashion (categories) was analysed at one and two years, and eleven years after bereavement, for each data source (Tables 5, 6 and 7). The first 24 months were examined, as it was during this period that the majority of new illnesses occurred (Table 4). A formal analysis of individual diseases in each category could not be done due to the very small numbers of individual diseases. Individual diseases listed as 'increased' in this section were those which appeared to the authors to be elevated among bereaved and possibly responsible for the statistically significant increase observed in the ICD-9 category.

During the first twelve months following the event, bereaved spouses reported a statistically significant excess of disorders in three categories: circulatory, mental, and respiratory disorders (Tables 5, 6, 7). Within the circulatory system category, angina and essential hypertension were increased for the bereaved (in all three sources of morbidity). Mental disorders which appeared to be increased were: anxiety state, neurotic depression, and depressive disorders not otherwise classified from the self-report morbidity source, and neurotic depression only from the record and confirmed morbidity sources. Diseases of the respiratory system category were increased in the self-report source only (Table 5). This increase appeared to be due to more cases of chronic sinusitis and bronchitis in the bereaved.

At two years post-bereavement, circulatory as well as psychiatric disorders showed a stadstically significant increase in the bereaved compared with the non-bereaved according to all three morbidity sources (Tables 5, 6 and 7). The diseases which were increased in each of these categories were those originating in the first year, and remaining prevalent into the second year. After two years of bereavement, the self-report and confirmed morbidity sources also showed a statistically significant increase in the number of diseases grouped under the respiratory and musculoskeletal categories.

At full follow-up time, combining the results of the three morbidity sources, eight of the seventeen ICD-9 categories showed a statistically significantly greater increase in morbidity rate in the bereaved compared with the controls. These categories were: circulatory; mental; neoplasms; endocrine, nutritional and metabolic; injury; digestive; respiratory and musculo-skeletal. In the circulatory system category, the diseases showing an increase were essential hypertension and angina, in all three sources of morbidity. The main diseases showing an increase in the mental disorders category were: neurotic depression, and depressive disorders not classified elsewhere (in all three morbidity sources), substance abuse (in the self-report and record sources), and reactive confusion (in the record morbidity data only).

Diseases in the other categories were also examined up to 11 years after bereavement. Skin neoplasia was reported (self-report data), but this appeared to be due to an increase in hyperkeratoses when doctors files were reviewed. Respiratory disorders were increased and, as with the one and two year follow-up results, the diseases which appeared to be increased were chronic sinusitis and bronchitis. Diseases which could be grouped under degenerative arthritides appeared increased in the musculo-skeletal system and those grouped under upper gastro-intesdnal tract disorders were increased in the digestive system. For the other two ICD-9 categories which were found to be higher in the bereaved (injury and endocrine, nutritional and metabolic), no particular disease appeared increased, rather the overall combined number of various diseases in the category was responsible for the observed increase of the category.

Overall, only two ICD-9 categories were consistently elevated at one, two and 11 years follow-up in the bereaved for all morbidity sources. These were: diseases of the Circulatory System (Category VII) and Mental Disorders (Category V). The respiratory system category (chronic sinusitis and bronchitis) was consistently elevated at one, two years and full follow-up time only in the self report source. It should be emphasised that the psychiatric and cardiovascular increases were found in all three data sources.

Numbers of diseases in each ICD-9 categories were too low to allow an examination of potential confounders (Table 1) in each ICD-9 category.

PATTERNS OF INCREASED MORBIDITY
There are three possible ways to explain the increased morbidity observed, and these are not mutually exclusive. Firstly, there could be more bereaved subjects ill than non-bereaved. It was found that, for all three sources of morbidity data, fewer bereaved subjects remained well throughout the follow-up period when compared with the controls. In the self-

Table 8. Number of illnesses per subject at full follow-up time (among subjects with at least 1 illness).

Number of Illnesses

Sources of data	Bereaved Median	IQR[1]	Controls Median	IQR[1]	p-value[2]
Self-Report	5	3, 6.5	4	2, 6	0.05
Record	6	4, 9.5	6	3, 8	0.3
Confirmed	2	1, 3.0	1	0, 3	0.4

1 - Interquartile Range
2 - Wilcoxin Rank Sum Test

report source 1% of bereaved subjects were illness-free during the follow-up dme compared with 13% for controls. For the record source these percentages were 1% for bereaved compared with 5% for controls, and for the confirmed source, 24% compared with 33%.

Secondly, of those subjects who were ill, there could have been more diseases per subject in the bereaved group than in the control group. This did not occur to any substantial degree (Table 8).

Thirdly, of those subjects who were ill, the bereaved could have suffered more long-term illnesses (which have a greater contribution to the overall illness-score morbidity measure) than the nonbereaved. This did occur. For example, in the confirmed morbidity source there were ten illnesses of bereaved subjects which lasted the full 11 years follow-up (ie. 110 illness-score) compared with four among the controls (44 illness-score). A higher percentage of illness among the non-bereaved was short-term (Table 9) and these contributed little to the total illness-score for the controls.

Table 9. Number of short-term[1] illnesses in bereaved compared with controls

	Bereaved			Controls		
Morbidity Data Source	Number of Short-Term Illnesses n	%	Total Illnesses	Number of Short-Term Illnesses n	%	Total Illnesses
Self-Report	162	46.2	351	160	49.8	322
Record	306	61.7	496	359	72.4	496
Confirmed	67	43.5	154	74	50.7	146

1 - short-term: an illness of up to, and including one year duration

The above results led to the examination of an hypothesis that bereaved who suffered high levels of early morbidity would be those who also suffered high levels of late morbidity. Conversely, bereaved with low levels of morbidity would also have low levels later on. Early morbidity episodes were defined as those occurring up to, and including, two years of follow-up, while late episodes were those between five and 11 years inclusive. In the early or late period, as appropriate, bereaved with a 'high' level of morbidity were those who had a umber of illness-years which was more than the average for controls, plus one standarddeviation. All other bereaved were considered to have a 'low' level of morbidity by default. The results show that the health status of individuals in the first two years after bereavement is related to their health status in the period five to 11 years after bereavement. Individuals who suffered a high level of morbidity after bereavement are still likely to be suffering high levels later (Table 10); the converse is also observed. Although, in some cases, the relative morbidity rates decrease between two years and full follow-up time (Tables 5-7) the majority

Table 10. **Bereaved** subjects and their health status in time

Morbidity data source	Percent of bereaved subjects who had the same level of morbidity early[1] and late[2] in the follow-up period	
	Low level of morbidity[3]	High level of morbidity[3]
Self-report	80.4%	57.7%
Record	71.7%	65.4%
Confirmed	83.7%	60.9%

1 - early: up to 2 years after bereavement
2 - late: between 5 years after bereavement and full follow-up time
3 - high and low levels of morbidity are defined as above and below the mean number of illnesses for the controls

remain substantial and statistically significant.

V. DISCUSSION

In this study, the morbidity of bereaved, up to 11 years after the event, has been examined. This morbidity was collected in two ways to ensure data quality: firstly, using subjects reports on their illnesses, and secondly, using records, either doctors data cards or hospital records as required. The data obtained allowed categorisation of the data by ICD-9 code and subsequent analysis. Currently, this work is unique and it will therefore not always be possible to discuss the results in the context of other research.

Bereaved subjects fared worse than control subjects in terms of their health (Table 2). However, although the two original sources (self-report and record reports) indicate similar relative elevations in morbidity rate, they apparently refer to different illnesses. The rate of disease agreement between the two sources was examined and found to be low for both bereaved and controls. This low confirmation rate could reflect that 'confirmation' of an illness required both temporal agreement between subject and record sources as well as agreement in the description of the disorder. It is possible that the large number of unconfirmed illnesses are in part caused by differences in timing between the subject's recollection of occurrence of the disease and their visit to the doctor. Most importantly though, this is an indication that bereaved subjects are not simply exaggerating their illnesses; after matching of the two sources, there are 'extra' diseases in the medical record source as well as the self-report source for both bereaved and non-bereaved alike.

The comparatively low numbers of illnesses which were reported by both subjects and medical practitioners (ie. the confirmed source) resulted in a relatively low statistical power in this source. Hence the fewer times that statistically significant results were found in that source when compared with the two original sources. When interpreting the results of confirmed reports, one must bear in mind that this source is derived from two 'real' sources. Thus although it is in one sense a reliable source, since there can be little doubt that confirmed illnesses did occur, it is also likely to substantially under-state the true number of illnesses.

It should be noted that twelve subjects originally enrolled as bereaved subjects were not reenrolled for this study (11 refused and one lost), compared with only one control who refused and one lost. If this differential recruitment rate has biased the results in any way, it is likely to have reduced the number of illnesses found in the bereaved, since the bereaved who refused did not have good health outcomes as discussed in the Method section, 'Subjects'.

The ICD-9 system categories, at one and two years, were examined for the three data sources (self report, medical record and confirmed). An increase in diseases within the mental category of the ICD-9 code in the first two years in all data sources was predictable, and consistent with other research.[2,3,21-29] However the size of the increase was surprising: for example a 3.7 fold increase in mental disorders in the bereaved at two years after bereavement (confirmed data source). The relative morbidity rate for the cardiovascular system was also elevated in the bereaved in the first two years. This appeared to be comprised mainly of essential hypertension and angina, and again the size of the increases was impressive: for example, a 3.5 fold increase in the bereaved at two years after the event (record source). Lastly, occurring only in the self-report source, respiratory disorders (chronic sinusitis and bronchitis) were increased in the bereaved in the first two years as were musculo-skeletal illnesses at two years. It is quite understandable that such respiratory diseases and degenerative arthritides may not be found in the record morbidity source because of a relatively more trivial perception of such illness, and thus subjects may not have sought medical advice. This should not put in question the existence of such disorders. It should also be noted that the increase in repiratory disease self-reporting soon after bereavement coincides with the literature reports[6,30] of depressed immune function and increased infectious illness rates in association with psychosocially distressing circumstances.

No other study is available for comparison with the results of the full follow-up ICD-9 category analysis. The increase in mental disorders at full follow-up is notable (for example, 2.1 fold increase in the bereaved in the record source) and may reflect poor resolution of bereavement issues so many years later. Increases were also found for respiratory and musculo-skeletal disorders (self report data only). The cardiovascular findings at full follow-up are surprising by their existence and by the size of the increase: for example 2.0 fold increase in the bereaved according to the record source. Various mechanisms can be postulated to explain these latter results. The medical literature has reflected an increasing interest (even priority) in the understanding of psychosomatic mechanisms in the pathogenesis of hypertension,[31] emphasising the importance of neurohumoral responses in the presumed defense reaction. Acute stress may operate via neural mechanisms, ie stimulated cardiac sympathetic nerves to the production of coronary artery spasm, angina pectoris and myocardial ischaemia and conduction disorders.[32] However, studies by Steptoe[33] have led to cautious interpretation of the catecholamine hypothesis. Another possible chronic stress mechanism might operate through neurogenic pathways to the development of hypertension.[34] The links between bereavement stress, hypertension and coronary thrombosis could operate via damaged intimal surfaces, platelet activation and increased circulating plasma lipids. Animal studies do confirm a link between stress and elevated free fatty acids.[35]

Explanations for the overall increase in morbidity observed were also sought. It appeared to be due to a combination of two factors. Firstly, more bereaved subjects were ill than controls. This is not surprising as the loss of a spouse is considered to be one of the most stressful life events.[36] Future work will investigate whether the increase observed is due to an early onset of morbidity (ie. morbidity which would have occurred naturally later in time) or additional morbidity.

Secondly, it was also found that, not only did more bereaved become ill following bereavement, but that their illnesses were of longer duration, and further, that their health status in the first few years following bereavement was associated with their health status 5 to 11 years later. These are more surprising results, perhaps not as much for the long-term psychiatric sequelae, as for the long-term increased physical morbidity.

In the current study none of the factors listed in Table 1 explained the effect of bereavement. When adjustments were made for factors listed in Table 1, particularly those found to be unequally distributed between bereaved and non-bereaved which included measures of SES[37] and marital status, it was concluded that none of these factors biased the comparison of bereaved and control morbidity rates. The one factor for which there was some evidence of a potential bias, the taking of medication on a chronic basis, may be a confounding variable or itself a result of the original bereavement stress and thus an outcome rather than a confounder. As well, it must be considered that in performing the confounder analysis the number of comparisons performed was 16 (variables in Table 1) x 3 (data sources). Thus, any apparent confounding must also be viewed in the context that the large number of comparisons performed increases the chance of finding an apparent confounding relationship, even when one does not truly exist. It should be noted that while we believe that the factors examined in this study represent a comprehensive investigation of potential confounders, there is always the possibility that some critical factor was not addressed. For example, dietary factors could not be measured in this study. Further, work is continuing on factors measured at the time of bereavement in 1975, 1976 or 1977 such as psychosocial factors including access of the bereaved to help and support from nuclear relatives and close friends, and certain biological variables such as tests of immunological function and their potential for predicting the morbidity results obtained here.

VI. CONCLUSION

It is believed that there is a psychological grieving process, in which, eventually, grief resolution occurs in most cases.[38-40] However, there is a wide range of symptoms associated with grief and there is no consensus as to what is considered a 'normal' process and what is 'unresolved grief'. Further, the time of resolution between individuals appears to vary greatly although overall, more bereaved become well adjusted to widowhood over time.[39,40] The results presented in this paper do add a new dimension to the grief process: long-term physical health sequelae. It is one thing to eventually achieve grief resolution and another to be left with a long-term health sequel which, from our data, appears to occur largely in the first few years following bereavement.

Pieces of the puzzle are still missing. It is not known who suffers increased long-term morbidity. Is it those at risk of a poor outcome (resolution)? Is it those who have 'unresolved grief' for a longer time? Is increased morbidity present as long as there is 'unresolved grief'? Is bereavement a risk factor for increased long-term morbidity irrespective of grief resolution? There is good evidence that grief support has been beneficial to the grieving process, certainly for individuals at risk of a poor resolution.[38,41,42] Is grief support also beneficial to, and does it help reduce, the long-term physical health sequelae? With more studies[43] establishing links between psychological response to diseases and prognosis, it could very well be that the answer to this last question is yes.

The questions mentioned above and other related issues still have to be answered. Bereavement is a life event with a high incidence and prevalence; it has been associated with long-term psychological and, now, important long-term physical adversity. This increase is not only of obvious consequence to the quality of life of these individuals, but also of importance in its costs to society, specifically, in terms of medical and community support expenses and absenteeism from work. Finding an answer to these questions is of paramount importance in human and financial terms.

VII. REFERENCES

1. *Population and Housing Census*, Australian Government Publishing Service, Canberra, 1986.
2. Parkes, C.M., Psychosomatic effects of bereavement, in *Modern Trends in Psychosomatic Medicine*, Hill, O.W., Ed., Butterworths, London, 1970. 71.
3. Klerman, G.L. and Izen, J.E., The effects of bereavement and grief on physical health and general wellbeing, in *Psychosomatic Medicine*, Reichsman, F., Ed., Karger, Basel, 1977. 63.
4. McAvoy, B.R., Death after bereavement, *Br.Med.J.*, 293, 835, 1986.
5. Rogers, M.P. and Reich, P., On the health consequences of bereavement. Editorial, *New Eng.J.Med.*, 319, 510, 1988.
6. Bartrop, R.W., Luckhurst, E., Lazarus, L.D., Kiloh, L.G. and Penny, R., Depressed lymphocyte function after bereavement, *Lancet*, 1, 834, 1977.
7. Bartrop, R.W., Stress and bereavement: a model for disease ? in *Advances in Behavioural Medicine*, Sheppard, J.L., Ed., Cumberland College of Health Sciences, Sydney, 1981. 85.
8. Porritt, D.W. and Bartrop, R.W., The independence of pleasant and unpleasant affect: the effects of bereavement, *Aust.J.Psychol.*, 37, 205, 1985.
9. Bartrop, R.W. and Porritt, D.W., The biological sequelae of adverse experiences, in *Handbook of Social Psychiatry*, Henderson, A.S. and Burrows, G.D., Eds., Elsevier, Amsterdam, 1988. 149.
10. Schleifer, S.J., Keller, S.E., Camerino, M., Thornton, J.C. and Stein, M., Suppression of lymphocyte stimulation following bereavement, *J.A.M.A.*, 250, 374, 1983.

11. Irwin, M., Daniels, M., Risch, S.C., Bloom, E. and Weiner, H., Plasma cortisol and natural killer cell activity during bereavement, *Biol.Psychiatry*, 24, 173, 1988.

12. *Australian Veterans Health Studies. Pilot study report*, Australian Government Publishing Service, Canberra, 1983.

13. Bartrop, R.W., Penny, R. and Forcier, L., Grief, immunity, morbidity and mortality: psychophysiological interactions, in *On the Inside of Illness*, Engelman, S., Ed., Irvington Press, New York, 1991. In press.

14. Snedecor, G.W. and Cochran, W.G., *Statistical Methods*, 7th ed., Ames: Iowa State Univ. Press, 1982.

15. Connover, W.J., *Practical Nonparametic Statistics*, 2nd ed., Wiley, New York, 1980.

16. Breslow, N.E., Lubin, J.E., Marek, P. and Langholtz, B., Multiplicative Models and Cohort Analysis, *JASA*, 78, 1, 1983.

17. Dixon, W.J., Brown, M.B., Engelman, L., Hill, M.A. and Jennerich, R.I., *BMDP Statistical Software Manual Vols 1 & 2*, Univ.Cal.Press, Berkeley, 1988.

18. McNeil, D.R. and Lunn, D., *SPIDA User's Manual*, Southwood Press, Sydney, 1988.

19. Baker, R.J. and Nelder, J.A., *The GLIM System-release*, Oxford Numerical Algorithms Group, 1978.

20. World Health Organisation, *International Classification of Diseases*, 9th ed., Geneva, 1975.

21. Schmale, A., Relationship of separation and depression in disease, *Psychosom.Med.*, 20, 259, 1958.

22. LeShan, L. and Worthington, R.E., Loss of cathexes as a common psychodynamic characteristic of cancer patients. An attempt at statistical validation of a critical hypothesis, *Psychol.Rep.*, 2, 183, 1958.

23. Parkes, C.M., Effects of bereavement on physical and mental health. A study of the medical records of widows, *Br.Med.J.*, 11, 274, 1964.

24. Parkes, C.M. and Brown, R., Health after bereavement. A controlled study of young Boston widows and widowers, *Psychosom.Med.*, 34, 449, 1972.

25. Maddison, D.C. and Viola, A., The health of widows in the year following bereavement, *J.Psychosom.Res.*, 12, 297, 1968.

26. Heyman, D.K. and Gianturco, D.T., Long-term adaptation by the elderly to bereavement, *J.Gerontol.*, 28, 359, 1973.

27. Clayton, P.J., Mortality and morbidity in the first year of widowhood, *Archs Gen.Psychiatry*, 125, 747, 1974.

28. Clayton, P.J., The sequelae and non-seqelae of conjugal bereavement, *Am.J.Psychiatr.*, 136, 1530, 1979.

29. Thompson, L.W., Breckenridge, J.N., Gallagher, D. and Peterson, J., Effects of bereavement on self perceptions of physical health in elderly widows and widowers, *J.Gerontol.*, 39, 309, 1984.

30. Jemmott, J.B. and Locke, S.E., Psychosocial factors, immunological investigation and human susceptibility to infectious diseases: how much do we know ? *Psychol.Bull.*, 95, 78, 1984.

31. Esler, M., Jennings, G., Komer, P. and et al., Assessment of human sympathetic nervous system activity from measurements of norepinephrine turnover, *Hypertension*, 3, 20, 1988.

32. Lown, B., Desilva, R.A., Reich, P. and Murawski, B.J., Psychophysiologic factors

in sudden cardiac death, *Am.J.Psychiatr.*, 137, 1325, 1980.

33. Steptoe, A., Renewal of interest in studies of personality, psychophysiology and symptomatology in essential hypertension, *J.Psychosom.Res.*, 27, 85, 1983.

34. Shapiro, D. and Goldstein, I., Behavioural patterns as they relate to hypertension, in *Clinical Pathophysiology of Arterial Hypertension*, Rosenthal, J., Ed., Springer, New York, 1983.

35. Bassett, J.R., Psychological stress and the coronary artery in ischaemic heart disease, in *The Coronary Artery*, Kalsner, S., Ed., Croom Helm, London, 1982. 474.

36. Holmes, T.H. and Rahe, R.H., The social readjustment rating scale, *J.Psychosom.Res.*, 11, 213, 1967.

37. Marmot, M.G., Kogevinas, M. and Elston, M.A., Social/economic status and disease, *Ann.Rev.Public Health*, 8, 111, 1987.

38. Windholz, M.J., Marmar, C.R. and Horowitz, M.J., A review of the literature on conjugal bereavement: impact on health and efficacy of intervention, *Compr.Psychiatry*, 26, 433, 1985.

39. Zisook, S. and Shuchter, S.R., The first four years of widowhood, *Psychiat.Annals*, 16, 288, 1986.

40. Middleton, W. and Raphael, B., Bereavement: State of the art and state of the science, *Psych.Clin.N.Amer.*, 10, 329, 1987.

41. Raphael, B., Preventive intervention with the recently bereaved, *Archs Gen.Psychiatry*, 34, 1450, 1977.

42. Parkes, C.M., Bereavement counselling: does it work? *Br.Med.J.*, 281, 3, 1980.

43. O'Donnell, M., Silove, D. and Wakefield, D., Current perspectives on immunology and psychiatry, *Aust.N.Z.J.Psychiatry*, 22, 366, 1988.

WHY DOES MODERATE EXERCISE ENHANCE, BUT INTENSE TRAINING DEPRESS, IMMUNITY ?

John A. Smith, Scott J. McKenzie, Richard D. Telford[a] and Maurice J. Weidemann

Department of Biochemistry, Faculty of Science, The Australian National University, Canberra, ACT, 2601, and [a]The Australian Institute of Sport, P.O. Box 176, Belconnen, ACT, 2616, Australia.

I. ABSTRACT

Neutrophil microbicidal activity was assessed in untrained and highly-trained male subjects (n=9,11) before and after one hour of cycling at 60% of maximum aerobic capacity. Luminol-enhanced chemiluminescence was monitored to peak intensity following stimulation with opsonized zymosan (OZ) (5-500 particles/cell) and, in untrained subjects only, their ability to kill opsonized *Staphylococcus aureus* was assessed by following the green (living) to red (dead) transition of acridine orange-stained bacteria by fluorescence microscopy. Irrespective of training status, exercise caused significant "priming" of neutrophils to produce H_2O_2 and HOCl upon stimulation with OZ (p < 0.01). Killing capacity was also primed and this correlated with increased phagocytosis (p < 0.01). Compared to untrained individuals, neutrophil oxidative activity of trained subjects was depressed about 50% at low (unit) OZ concentration (p < 0.075) but not at saturation. The training trend was confirmed by a longitudinal study conducted over a 15 month period. Changes in the circulating concentrations of monokines (IL-1β and TNF-α) were too small, and built up too slowly, to account for the increased neutrophil respiratory burst activity. Observations from other laboratories showing that growth hormone, and possibly prolactin, are potent macrophage-priming agents suggest that these pituitary hormones may also trigger exercise-induced priming of neutrophils. Growth hormone undergoes a 10-fold change in plasma concentration in response to relatively mild exercise intensities below 65% of VO_{2max} that are insufficient to induce ACTH secretion; above this threshold, however, ACTH release triggered, possibly, by IL-1β and TNF-α interaction with pituitary or hypothalamic cells, may induce the release of immunosuppressive glucocorticoids and opioids into the circulation. If prolonged by regular training, elevated cortisol may have chronically depressive effects on immunity.

II. INTRODUCTION

This work began in 1987 after conversations we had with colleagues at the Australian Institute of Sport on the frequency with which elite athletes in training experience upper respiratory tract infections, particularly during the critical "taper" period immediately before a major competition. Could there be, we wondered, a connection between regular intensive training and depressed immunity? And, as the obverse of this, could there be - at a lower exercise intensity - a positive effect of moderate exercise on immunity that might raise resistance to common infections? There had been reports in the literature suggesting that separate episodes of moderate aerobic exercise might enhance immunity whilst intensive training might have chronic immunosuppressive effects.[1]

At the time we were struck by two observations - from unrelated sources - which suggested how the phenomena of physical exertion and altered immune cell reactivity might be connected. (i) Cannon & Kluger had shown, in 1983, that cycling for one hour at 60% of maximum capacity raised the circulating concentrations of "pyrogenic" agents in the blood of human subjects;[2] and (ii) a group of South African workers had demonstrated the presence of significant free endotoxin in the plasma of subjects at the end of an ultra marathon road race.[3] We knew also, from several isolated reports, that interleukin-1 and tumour necrosis factor, in particular - both of which are pyrogenic - have a variety of potential immunostimulatory effects. We originally hypothesized (Fig. l) that exercise may induce "priming" of neutrophils, and enhance their microbicidal activity, through the activities of

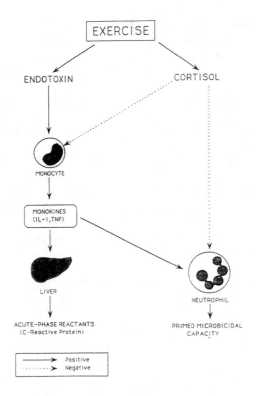

Figure 1. Proposed relationship between exercise and the modulation of neutrophil microbicidal activity by monokines and cortisol.

monokines (eg. interleukin-1β, tumour necrosis factor) that are released into the circulation following moderate exercise.[2] This might be attributable, in turn, to the "leakage" of small amounts of endotoxin from the mildly hypoxic gut into the portal circulation, as endotoxin is one of the most potent stimuli of pyrogen secretion from monocytes. Depressed neutrophil activity, on the other hand, is likely to be mediated through immunosuppressive glucocorticoids like cortisol which are released into the circulation to act as a counter-balancing negative signal once exercise reaches a critical intensity.

III. MATERIALS AND METHODS

MATERIALS

Sterile Hank's balanced salt solution containing 5mM D-glucose (HBSS) and phosphate buffered saline (PBS) were prepared by conventional methods. Luminol was prepared as a chemiluminogenic indicator by suspending 10 mg of luminol (5-amino-2,3-dihydro-1,4-phthalazine dione) (Boehringer, Mannheim, FRG) in 5ml of PBS containing 8mM triethylamine. The mixture was sonicated for 1 minute and shaken to give a clear solution. A single batch of opsonized zymosan (used for all experiments) was prepared by incubating 10 mg of Zymosan-A particles (highly glycosylated fragments of yeast cell walls) (Sigma. St Louis, MO:) with 1 ml of fresh human plasma for 30 min at 37°C. The suspension was centrifuged at 400 x g for 2 minutes and the pellet washed twice in PBS before resuspension at a final concentration of 10 mg/ml. Aliquots (1ml) were stored frozen and used only once after thawing. Counting by haemocytometer revealed that this preparation contained approx. 106 zymosan particles/microlitre.

HUMAN SUBJECTS

For the cross-sectional experiment, 9 healthy untrained male subjects (average VO_{2max} 48.1 ml/kg + 9, average age 22 years) and 11 elite male cyclists (average VO_{2max} 71.4 ml/kg $\pm$ 6, average age 19 years) were recruited. No subject had experienced symptoms of acute illness or had taken medication for 6 weeks prior to the test. The majority of the cyclists were competing at Australian national standard and maintained an intensive training regime of at least 25 hours/week. In contrast, all untrained subjects devoted less than 3 hours/week to exercise related activities. The project was approved by the Ethics in Human Experimentation Committee of the Australian National University. All subjects signed a consent form that described the aims of the project and its attendant risks. For the longitudinal experiment, 5 initially untrained males (16-18 years) selected to take part in an intensive rowing training program at the Australian Institute of Sport were used. Details of the subjects, their training regime and other parameters will be published elsewhere.

DETERMINATION OF VO_{2MAX}

Prior to the experimental testing period, the maximum rate of oxygen uptake (i.e. VO_{2MAX}) was determined for each individual by subjecting them to a progressive increase in work load to voluntary exhaustion on a cycle ergometer (Exertech, Melbourne, Vic.). A work monitor unit (Exertech, Melbourne, Vic) containing a magnetic sensor located close to a 60-tooth cog mounted on the front wheel generated a continuous analogue display of power output in watts (W). The initial power output was 50 W, and this was stepped up by increments of 25 W at each min. The subjects breathed through a one-way valve (Hans Rudolph 2700, Kansas City, MO) and the volume of air inspired was measured with a Morgan ventilation meter (Medox, Melbourne, Vic). Samples of inspired air were drawn continuously through a desiccant ($CaCl_2$) into oxygen and carbon dioxide analysers (Applied Electrochemistry, Sunnyvale, CL) calibrated against gravimetric standards.

Electrocardiograms (ECG) recorded during the final 10 seconds of each minute were transferred to an ECG computer (Quinton Instruments. Seattle. WA). Outputs from the ventilation meter, gas analysers and ECG computer were monitored by a LSI 11/21 computer (Digital Electrical Corporation, Sydney, N.S.W.) programmed to give minute-by-minute readouts of pulmonary ventilation at standard temperature and pressure for dry gas (STPD). Oxygen uptake, carbon dioxide output, respiratory exchange ratio, heart rate and ventilatory equivalents for oxygen (VO_2) and carbon dioxide (VCO_2) were recorded for each subject.

EXERCISE PROTOCOL

A standardized exercise schedule was undertaken by each subject. Food intake before the test was restricted to a light "non-fatty" meal. The experiments were carried out in the morning (i.e. 9.30-10.30 am) to take advantage of the overnight rest: some additional experiments were performed in the afternoon (i.e. 3.30-4.30 pm) to test for circadian variation in neutrophil oxidative activity. No other strenuous activity was undertaken throughout the 24 hour period. All subjects exercised on a cycle ergometer (Exertech, Melbourne, Vic) for one hour at a work output equivalent to 60% of their individually-determined values. This workload is sufficient to elevate the circulating endogenous pyrogen activity of human subjects.[2] The power output was monitored with a work monitor unit (Exertech, Melbourne, Vic). Blood samples were taken by venipuncture (arm anticubital vein) immediately before (i.e. at rest) and after exercise. A third sample was taken 6 hours later to check for the persistence of exercise induced changes.

PREPARATION OF NEUTROPHILS

Heparinized blood (10ml) was decanted onto a 3ml Ficol-paque cushion (Pharmacia, Uppsala, Sweden) in a 15 ml sterile tube and centrifuged for 15 minutes at 600 x g. The neutrophil layer was removed from the top of the red blood cell layer by aspiration and transferred to a second sterile tube. Contaminating red blood cells were removed by hypotonic shock with 0.83% NH_4Cl. The mixture was centrifuged at 400 x g for 5 minutes. The cell pellet was washed twice in 0.83% NH4Cl to remove residual red blood cells and then resuspended in HBSS. The suspension was stored on ice before use. The purity of the cell preparation, checked by differential staining with Harclo "diff-quik" (Lab-Aids, Sydney, N.S.W.), was greater than 95% neutrophils, of which more than 95% excluded trypan blue.

CHEMILUMINESCENCE

The productdon of reactive oxygen species by 105 neutrophils in response to stimulation with opsonized zymosan in the concentration range 5-500 particles/cell was estimated by measuring the chemiluminescence generated by the co-oxidation of luminol by the hydrogen peroxide and hypochlorous acid produced by the cells; it is a measure of "true phagocytosis", since the release of myeloperoxidase activity, which generates $HOCl^-$, requires azurophilic degranulation. Chemiluminescence was measured in a 1251 Luminometer (LKB Wallac, Turku, Finland) at 37^0 with continuous stirring of the reaction mixture. Neutrophils suspended in HBSS were added to polystyrene luminometer tubes (Clinicon 2174-086 Turku, Finland) containing 900ml of HBSS and luminol (113 μM).The reaction mixture was preincubated for 5 min to determine baseline chemiluminescence. Opsonized zymosan was then added to give a total volume of 1.0 ml. The chemiluminescence signal [expressed in millivolts (mV)]was recorded continuously up to peak velocity on an LKB 2210 potentiometric chart recorder (LKB-produkter AB, Bromma, Sweden).

STATISTICAL ANALYSIS

Wilcoxon's sum rank test and Student's t-test were used to assess the significance of differences attributable to either training or acute exercise (i.e. untrained/trained; rested/exercised; rested/six hours post-exercise; and exercised/six hours post-exercise). Non-parametric methods were used to check the values arrived at using Student 's t-test. The significance levels obtained independently agreed quite closely in most cases. Where data are presented as means + SEM, the significance of the differences claimed is based on the larger value obtained from the two tests.

IV. RESULTS

In the first experiment we compared, before and after exercise, the respiratory burst activities of neutrophils isolated from highly-trained elite athletes (20 year old male cyclists training 25 hours/week) with those from age-matched male undergraduates who regularly undertook less than three hours of exercise per week (the untrained control group). The experimental exercise regime tested each individual for one hour at 60% of his own, previously-determined, VO_{2max}. The parameter we chose to measure, initially, was the rate at which neutrophils produce cytotoxic, oxygen-centered free radicals in response to a phagocytic challenge, as this is one of the most sensitive indicators of whether the cells have been exposed to circulating pyrogens (or to some equivalent "priming" stimulus). To do this,

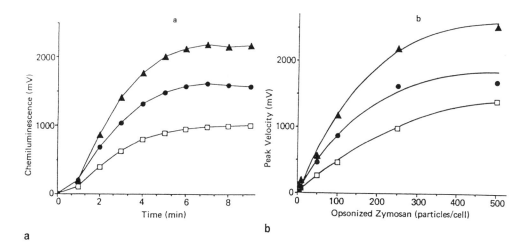

Figure 2. Effect of exercise on reactive oxygen production by zymosan-stimulated neutrophils: a typical individual response measured before (□), immediately after (▲) and six hours after exercise (○). (a) Time course following stimulation with opsonized zymosan (250 particles/cell). (b) Concentration dependence: peak chemiluminescence determined over a range of zymosan concentrations. (5-500 particles/cell). Reproduced from Smith *et al*[4] with permission of Georg Thieme Verlag, Stuttgart, New York.

we measured the rate of photon output generated by the cooxidation of luminol by H_2O_2 and hypochlorous acid during the respiratory burst. In both trained and untrained individuals, the cells recovered after moderate exercise responded to sdmulation with opsonized zymosan particles with an increased rate of free radical production, and they did so over the complete range of subsaturating and saturating particle concentrations (5-500/cell) (Fig. 2).

When these data were transformed and analysed (by log/log plot), the analysis yielded two useful kinetic constants (Fig. 3):

    (i)   the *intercept* on the y axis, which is indicative of the *specific rate of free radical production* (k) at unit stimulus concentration; and

    (ii)   the *slope* of the line, which is indicative of the order of the reaction.

For each individual tested, aerobic exercise consistently raised the value of the interceptindicating increased activity of the cells at low stimulus concentration-without altering the slope of the double logarithmic plot. Furthermore, the cells sustained this increased activity for at least 6 hours (Fig. 3).

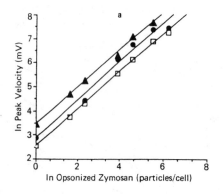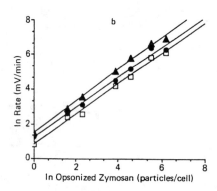

Figure 3. Determination of kinetic constants by analysis of data shown in Fig. 2. (a) Double logarithm plot of peak chemiluminescent velocity versus zymosan concentration; (b) Double logarithm plot of maximum rate of acceleration to peak chemiluminescence versus zymosan concentration. Reproduced from Smith *et al*[4] with permission of Georg Thieme Verlag, Stuttgart, New York.

The "box and whisker" plot shown in Fig. 4 contains the *individual values* of the intercept k for all subjects tested and compares the trained with the untrained group. In spite of the large spread of absolute values, paired statistical testing revealed that "the exercise effect" i.e. the sustained increase in the specific rate of free radical production for 6 hours - was highly significant in the trained and untrained groups alike; but, most surprisingly, the absolute values were severely depressed by training. These results, which have been published in full elsewhere,[4] indicate that the capacity of human neutrophils to produce microbicidal reactive oxygen species upon stimulation *in vitro* - under conditions that simulate a microbial challenge - is "primed" significantly in response to one hour of cycling at 60% of maximum aerobic capacity. Compared to untrained controls, the specific activity of the neutrophil oxidative burst is 50% lower, both before and after exercise, in subjects training intensively for 25 hours/week.

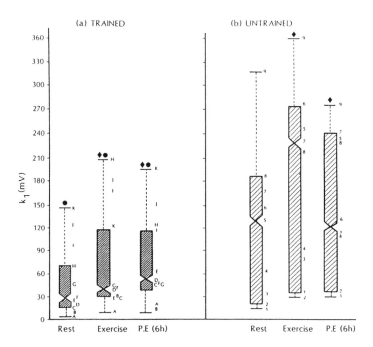

Figure 4. Effect of exercise and training on the kinetic constants (k_1) (peak CL velocity at unit particle concentration) determined by transforming the primary data obtained from each individual subject as shown in Fig. 2a. The "box and whisker" plot shows the individual values of k_1 (A-K for the trained and 1-9 for the untrained subjects) displayed for the resting, exercised, and 6 hour post-exercised states. The "box" by each data set contains the middle 50% of the values where half lie above the median (at the point of indentation) and half below it, and the dashed "whiskers" represent the upper and lower 25% extremities. Significant differences (Wilcoxon test): ($p < 0.01$) due to exercise ($\blacklozenge$); and ($p < 0.075$) due to training ($\circ$). Reproduced from Smith *et al*[4] with permission of Georg Thieme Verlag, Stuttgart, New York.

We followed up this cross-sectional study with a 15-month longitudinal study of 5 initially untrained males selected to take part in an intensive rowing training program at the Australian Institute of Sport. As shown in Fig. 5, the initially high "k" values for resting neutrophils were depressed progressively as training continued. The greatest fall occurred at the point where the training intensity increased abruptly (from 15 hours to 25 hours/week, with a corresponding increase in work intensity). The specific rate remained significantly depressed throughout the next four months of intensive training.

Longitudinal Study

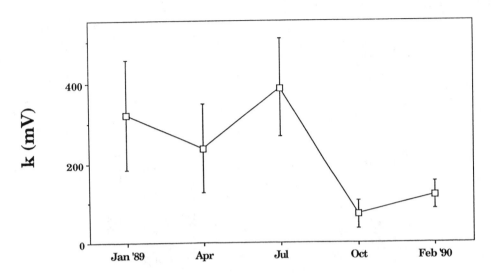

Figure 5. Results (means +SEM) of a longitudinal study showing the effect of training on kinetic constant k_1 determined with neutrophils isolated from 5 initially untrained male subjects (Jan 1989) undertaking a training schedule sufficient to bring them to national competitive standard in 15 months. The training intensity and frequency increased markedly (from 15-25 hours/week) between July and October 1989.

This initial study raised a number of related questions that were accessible to experimental investigation:

(a) *Is the exercise effect due to the release of trapped cells with intrinsically higher activity from marginated pools ?*

We know that the circulating white blood cell count doubles or trebles after exercise and that this phenomenon can be evoked equally by a prolonged period of moderate exercise or a short burst of anaerobic exercise to exhaustion. In the experiment described in Fig. 6 we compared the effects of these two exercise regimes and found that, in spite of very strong demargination, maximum anaerobic exertion for one minute depressed rather than activated the specific rate of free radical production by neutrophils from trained and untrained subjects. This, we believe, eliminates the possibility that the cells ejected from marginated pools are intrinsically more "activated" than their circulating couterparts.

(b) *Does the enhanced free radical production observed in cells after exercise have any functional significance? (i.e. Does it lead to an enhanced rate of uptake or killing of bacteria?)*

To test this hypothesis, phagocytosis and killing of opsonized *Staphylococcus aureus* were measured by following the uptake, and green to red transition (indicative of cell death),

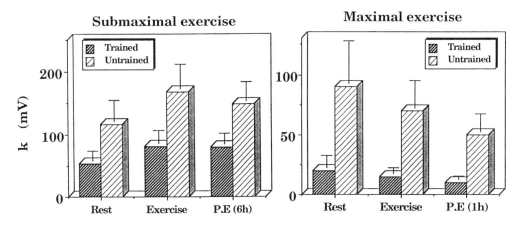

Figure 6. Comparison of the effect of submaximal (60 minutes at 60% VO_{2max}) and maximal exercise (1 minute at 100% VO_{2max}) on the value of kinetic constant k (peak CL velocity at unit particle concentration) determined at rest, immediately after exercise and at either one or six hours after exercise with neutrophils isolated from trained and untrained men.

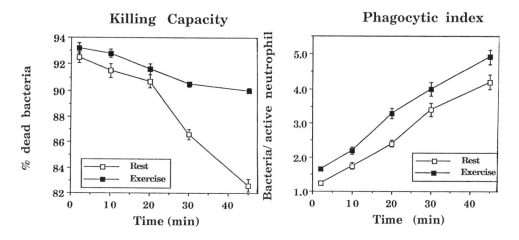

Figure 7. Effect of aerobic exercise on the phagocytic index (number of bacteria phagocytosed per active neutrophil) and killing capacity (% of dead bacteria present in actively phagocytosing neutrophils) of neutrophils isolated from untrained men. Monolayers of adherent neutrophils (on a glass coverslip) were prepared from 11 untrained men before and immediately after one hour of moderate exercise (60% VO_{2max}). Exercise did not change neutrophil adherence. Phagocytosis and killing of opsonized *Staphylococcus aureus* (added at 50 bacteria/cell) were determined by following the green (living) to red (dead) transition of acridine orange-stained bacteria by fluorescence microscopy.

of acridine orange-stained bacteria by fluorescence microscopy. Whilst exercise increased the total phagocytic activity per 100 cells, this was not due to an increase in the percentage of phagocytically-active cells, which confirms the conclusion we reached in the demargination experiment. Rather, as Fig. 7 shows, exercise increased the number of bacteria taken up per active neutrophil over the entire time course; and it prevented the rapid decline in bactericidal activity that we observed after 20 minutes in cells isolated from resting subjects.

    (c)   *Do recombinant pyrogenic cytokines have the same effect as exercise in "priming" neutrophils to produce free radicals at a higher rate?*

    Figure 8 shows that incubating cells isolated at rest with recombinant human tumour necrosis factor (TNF-α) for 20 minutes caused essentially the same kinetic response as 60 minutes of exercise: the intercepts were increased in each case without significant change of slope. Interleukin-1 had virtually the same effect as TNF, and the response obtained when the two cytokines were added together did not appear to be additive or potentiating.

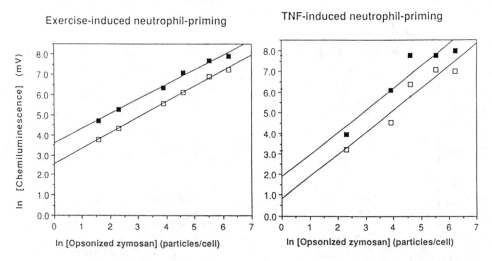

Figure 8. Comparison of the effect of exercise (60min at 60% VO_{2max}) and recombinant human TNF-α (5-10 pg/ml) on the kinetics of the chemiluminescent response of neutrophils to opsonized zymosan. The left hand panel shows that cells from exercised individuals (■) respond to opsonized zymosan with enhanced oxidative burst activity at unit stimulus concentration (determined from the intercept) compared with cells from the same individual at rest (□). The right hand panel shows that pretreatment of neutrophils from non-exercised subjects with recombinant TNF-α (5-10pg/ml) (■) for 30 min at 37°C before stimulation with opsonized zymosan produced, compared with untreated cells (□), a similar "priming" effect to that induced by exercise.

(d)   *Finally, we attempted to refine the early observations on exercise-induced pyrogen secretion by performing specific assays for TNF-α and IL-1β in the sera of resting and exercised individuals.*

Initially, using an ELISA, we found a relatively large but scattered exercise-induced increase in TNF-α in the majority of subjects. In attempting to confirm this with a more sensitive immunoradiometric assay, however, we found that the exercise-induced increases were much smaller, and were confined to the untrained individuals (result not shown). Likewise, using an immunoradiometric assay for IL-1β, we found a similar small, but significant, response to exercise, but this time the increase was confined to the trained subjects (p= 0.048). More importantly, however, the increases were not apparent immediately after aerobic exercise (60 min at 60% VO_{2max}) but appeared to require about six hours to reach the maximum value. In other words, the circulating concentrations of pyrogenic cytokines built up far too slowly after aerobic exercise to account for the rapid onset of neutrophil "priming". Even at six hours the circulating concentrations of IL-1 and TNF may be insufficient to trigger any enhancement of neutrophil microbicidal activity, but may contribute to maintaining the primed state if this has been initiated by an earlier stimulus.

Experiments carried out on the same subjects showed that aerobic exercise did not alter the plasma concentrations of the lymphokines interferon-γ and granulocyte-macrophage colony stimulating factor, both of which are known to prime neutrophils for enhanced microbicidal activity *in vitro*.

V. DISCUSSION

The interactions between the neuro-endocrine and immune systems in response to physical exertion bear a remarkable resemblance to those accompanying psychological stress. Table 1 shows, in particular, that there are striking changes induced by exercise in the circulating concentrations of a number of anterior pituitary hormones; and that the sequence in which these hormones appear in the circulation is related, in turn, to the intensity of the exercise load. The most striking (and most well-established) observation is that growth hormone undergoes a ten-fold change after very mild exercise indeed, and that it does so in the absence of any increase in ACTH until a threshold intensity of 65% of VO_{2max} is reached.[5] It is *only beyond this threshold* that ACTH released from the anterior pituitary signals a rise in circulating cortisol that sets in train the dampening, or suppression, of a number of immune cell functions.

Two other pieces of evidence are required, however, to complete the logic behind the assembly of this speculative jigsaw. The first observation, made by Keith Kelly's group in 1988,[6] is that growth hormone is a very potent potentiator, or "primer", of the respiratory burst in monocytes and macrophages and may, by analogy, do the same thing in other phagocytic cells like neutrophils. The key observation, using either native or recombinant porcine somatotropin to stimulate superoxide production by macrophages, is shown in Fig. 9 [reproduced from Edwards *et al*[6]]. Both growth hormone and prolactin are potent activators of a range of immune mechanisms, including antibody production, T-lymphocyte proliferation and phagocyte microbicidal responses.[7] Secondly, several groups have now reported,[8,9] using

Table 1. The effects of exercise of different intensities on the circulating concentrations[†] of growth hormone, prolactin, substance P, ACTH and cortisol.

FACTOR	PRE-EXERCISE	POST-EXERCISE (65% VO₂ max)	POST EXERCISE (80% VO₂ max)
Growth Hormone[#] (ng/ml)	3.1 ± 0.9	19.7 ± 7.5*	41.3 ± 15.9*
Prolactin[‡] (ng/ml)	10.5 ± 2.5	12.5 ± 3.5	
Substance P[‡] (nmol/ml)	5.2 ± 0.85	7.05 ± 1.05*	
ACTH[#] (pg/ml)	40 ± 15	50 ± 17	125 ± 20*
Cortisol[#] (mg/ml)	14.5 ± 1.5	14.8 ± 1.0	15.7 ± 1.3*

[†]The data collected in this table are derived from values quoted in the literature: notably those of [#] Farrell, Garthwaite and Gustafson (1983) (5) and [‡] Goldfarb, Hatfield, Armstrong and Potts (1990) (11)
* indicates statistically significant difference from the pre-exercise value.

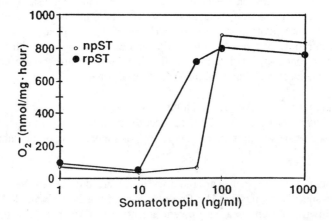

Figure 9. The effect of native, pituitary-derived porcine somatotropin (npST) and recombinant porcine somatotropin (rpST) on production of superoxide (O₂⁻) by porcine peripheral blood-derived mononuclear phagocytes. Cells were stimulated with opsonized zymosan after a 24 hour incubation with somatotropin. This figure is reproduced from Edwards *et al*[6] with permission of the authors and the publishers of Science.

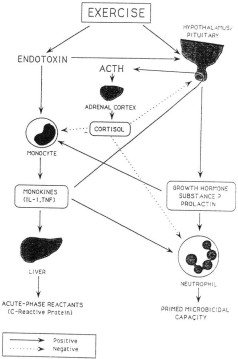

Figure 10. Proposed relationship between exercise, neuro-endocrine/cytokine changes and the microbicidal activity of neutrophils. The diagram shows how moderate exercise may induce "priming" of neutrophils through immunostimulatory pituitary hormones and/or an endotoxin-monokine cascade. Very intensive exercise may negate "priming" due to activation of the immunosuppressive arm of the pituitary adrenal axis. Reproduced from Smith *et al*[10] - by the present authors - with permission of the publisher of Medical Science Research (Elsevier Applied Science Publishers Ltd).

experimental animals, that IL-1β is a powerful stimulus of ACTH release from the anterior pituitary, which it may trigger, either directly, or via interaction with hypothalamic cells. Immunosuppressive effects might follow from the subsequent secretion of glucocorticoids and opioids that ACTH induces.

Figure 10 gathers together the disparate threads we have canvassed in this paper. It adds considerable detail to the rather simple cytokine model that we started out with (Fig. 1) and relates exercise, as a stressor, to the endocrinological features of the classical "stress response" that may compromise immunological function. We propose[10] that low to moderate levels of exercise may boost immunity through the action of growth hormone and, possibly, of prolactin and substance P, on a variety of cellular and humoral immune mechanisms. These beneficial effects may be negated once exercise intensity reaches a critical threshold and is sufficiently prolonged. The pivotal point where this occurs, at about 65% of maximum capacity, involves the triggering of ACTH release from the anterior pituitary in response to either direct stimulation by endotoxin released from gut-associated bacteria or, indirectly, via a rise in circulating monokines secondary to this event. ACTH, in turn, induces the release of immunosuppressive glucocorticoids and opioids into the circulation which, if prolonged, may have chronically depressive effects on immunity. While acute immunosuppression may prevent exercise-induced inflammatory injury, chronic depression of immune mechanisms, like those observed in some intensively-training athletes, may also increase susceptibility to infection.

This theoretical model may prove to be a useful framework for investigating the effects of stressors of different type and intensity on human immunity.[10]

VI. ACKNOWLEDGEMENTS

This work was supported by grants to Dr M.J.Weidemann from the Australian Research Grants Scheme and the Australian National University Faculties Research Fund. John A. Smith is a recipient of a Commonwealth Postgraduate Research Award. The authors wish to thank Mrs S. Niazi for typing the manuscript.

VII. REFERENCES

1. Fitzgerald, L., Exercise and the immune system, *Immunol.Today*, 9, 337, 1988.
2. Cannon, J.G. and Kluger, M.J., Endogenous pyrogen activity in human plasma after exercise, *Science*, 220, 617, 1983.
3. Bosenberg, A.T., Brock-Utne, J.G., Gaffin, S.L. and et al., , Strenuous exercise causes systemic endotoxemia, *J.Appl.Physiol.*, 65, 106, 1988.
4. Smith, J.A., Telford, R.D., Mason, I.B. and Weidemann, M.J., Exercise, training and neutrophil microbial activity, *Int.J.Sports Med.*, 11, 179, 1990.
5. Farrell, P.A., Garthwaite, T.L. and Gustafson, A.B., Plasma adrenocorticotropin and cortisol responses to submaximal and exhaustive exercise, *J.Appl.Physiol.*, 55, 1441, 1983.
6. Edwards, C.K.,III, Ghiasuddin, S.M., Schepper, J.M., Yunger, L.N. and Kelley, K.W., A newly defined property of somatotropin: Priming of macrophages for production of superoxide anion, *Science*, 239, 769, 1988.
7. Kelley, K.W., Growth hormone, lymphocytes and macrophages, *Biochem.Pharmacol.*, 38, 705, 1989.
8. Sapolsky, R., Rivier, C., Yamamoto, G., Plotsky, P. and Vale, W., Interleukin-1 stimulates the secretion of hypothalamic corticotropin-releasing factor, *Science*, 238, 522, 1987.
9. Bernton, E.W., beach, J.E., Holaday, J.W., Smallridge, R.C. and Fein, H.G., Release of multiple hormones by a direct action of interleukin-1 on pituitary cells, *Science*, 238, 519, 1987.
10. Smith, J.A. and Weidemann, M.J., *Med.Sci.Res.*, 18, 749, 1990.

EFFECTS OF EXERCISE DURING SPORTS TRAINING AND COMPETITION ON SALIVARY IgA LEVELS

L.T. Mackinnon, E. Ginn and G. Seymour[a]

Department of Human Movement Studies and [a]Department of Social and Preventive Dentistry andOral Biology, The University of Queensland, Brisbane, Queensland, 4072. Australia.

I. ABSTRACT

The high incidence of upper respiratory illness (URI) among competitive athletes has prompted studies on the effects of exercise on mucosal immunity. IgA, the major effector of mucosal immunity, has been shown to decrease following intense endurance exercise. Our current studies focus on mucosal immune function in elite Australian athletes.

Study 1 Salivary IgA was measured in samples obtained from 12 female hockey athletes before and after exercise during 3 training matches (low psychological stress) and 4 competitive matches over 5 days of major competition (high stress). Both pre- and post-exercise IgA concentrations (μg per ml saliva) were lower during competition compared to training (p < .001, 2 way ANOVA). IgA concentration (μg per mg salivary protein) declined after each exercise session during both training and competition. Both pre- and post-exercise IgA levels (μg per mg protein) declined progressively over the 5 days of competition.

Study 2 Salivary IgA flow rate was measured before and after 4 training sessions over 1 month in 8 male kayakers. IgA flow rate (μg per min) decreased after all sessions (p < .02, 2 way ANOVA). The largest decrease (51%) occurred during a session at the end of a week of especially intense training. Resting IgA concentration (μg per ml) was also lowest on this day.

Study 3 Of 14 male and female squash athletes followed over a 10 week period, 5 (36%) eshibited URI, as diagnosed by a physician. Saliva was collected before and after usual training on a weekly basis. In the athletes who became ill, 6 of the 7 occurrences of URI were preceeded (within 2 days) by exercise-induced decreases in IgA concentration (μg per ml) (p < .01, chi square analysis). Pre-exercise IgA levels were similar on days preceeding illness compared to all other days (means of 39.2 vs 39.1 μg per ml). However, mean IgA concentration decreased 22% (to 30.5 μg per ml) after exercise on days preceeding illness, while IgA levels increased (to 47.3 μg per ml) on all days not preceeding illness (p < .01, 1 way ANOVA on pre- to post- exercise differences). Taken together these data suggest that: (1) Psychological stress of sports competition may suppress mucosal immunity. (2) Reductions in both resting and post-exercise IgA levels may be cumulative during daily intense training and major competition. (3) There appears to be a temporal relationship between exercise-- induced decreases in IgA and subsequent URI.

II. INTRODUCTION

There is a general perception among elite athletes, their coaches and team physicians that athletes are susceptible to upper respiratory illness (URI) during intense sports training and major competiton.[1,2] This perception has been supported by epidemiological data. For example, up to 50% of runners completing a 56 km ultramarathon reported symptoms of URI turing the two weeks following the race, in contrast to only 15% of age- and gender-matched control subjects living in the same households as the runners. The incidence of illness increased as race time decreased (i.e. in the faster runners), and was higher in athletes who trained the hardest during the week prior to the race, suggesting an effect of exercise intensity.[3] In contrast, the incidence of URI has been reported to be lower in runners completing shorter races (21 km and less) compared to age- and gender-matched control subjects.[4] These data suggest that specific factors, such as fitness level and "competitiveness" of the athlete, as well as exercise intensity and duration have differing effects on mucosal immune function.

The high frequency of recurrent URI among elite athletes has prompted a number of recent studies on the effects of exercise on mucosal immune function, and especially IgA, the major immunoglobulin class in mucosal fluids.[2,5-9] Decreases in salivary IgA levels have been noted following intense endurance exercise in a variety of athletes, such as cross country skiers,[2] cyclists,[5,6] swimmers,[9] runners,[8] and hockey players.[7] It is currently unclear whether these declines in IgA levels observed after exercise are related to the increased incidence of URI in athletes.

Psychological stress has also been shown to decrease salivary IgA levels.[10] Elite competitive athletes experience significant physical stress of intense daily (often twice daily) exercise, as well as psychological stress associated with major competition. It is possible that there is a combined effect of psychological and physical stress associated with intense exercise during major competition in altering mucosal immunity to URI. The data presented here are part of ongoing work on the effects of exercise on mucosal immune function in elite Australian athletes. The work focuses on two basic questions: Firstly, does intense exercise alter mucosal immunity so that athletes are more susceptible to URI, and secondly, is the stress of competition additive to the effects of exercise in altering mucosal immunity?

III. METHODS

GENERAL

Three studies are reported below. For all studies, whole saliva was sampled immediately before and after exercise during either usual training or major sports competition. Saliva was immediately frozen and stored frozen until assayed for immunoglobulin (Ig) concentrations. Ig of interest were IgA, IgG and IgM, each of which was measured by.[11] For each Ig, a standard curve of knovn amounts of purified Ig (Dako) was run on each microtitre plate. To avoid interassay variability, all samples from each athlete were assayed on the same microtitre plate. Saliva protein concentration was measured by the standard Lowry assay.

STUDY 1 HOCKEY STUDY

Saliva was obtained from 12 female members of the Queensland Senior Women's Hockey Team before and after three training matches (low psychological stress) each spaced one week apart during the three weeks prior to the National Tournament, and then before and after four matches over a five day period during the National Tournament (high stress).

STUDY 2 KAYAK STUDY

Saliva was obtained from eight male members of the Australian Canoe Federation Kayak Unit before and after four regular training sessisns over a one month period. Timed samples were obtained, enabling a calculation of saliva flow rate and IgA flow rate.

STUDY 3 SQUASH STUDY

Saliva was obtained from 14 male and female members of the Australian Institute of Sport Squash Unit before and after regular training on a weekly basis over a ten week period. Athletes documented all illnesses during this period and reported to the team physician for a medical diagnosis.

IV. RESULTS AND DISCUSSION

STUDY 1 HOCKEY STUDY

Salivary IgA and IgM concentrations, espressed as μg Ig per ml saliva, were

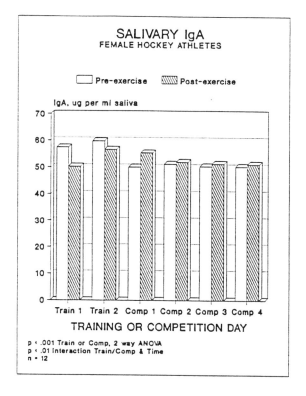

Figure 1. Salivary IgA concentration in female hockey athletes before and after two matches during training (Train) and four matches over five days of major competition (Comp). IgA levels were significantly lower (p < 0.01, 2-way ANOVA) during competition compared to training.

significantly lower (p < .001 for IgA and p < .01 for IgM) during competition compared to training (Figure 1 for IgA). The effect was most apparent for resting IgA and IgM concentrations. These data suggest that IgA and IgM, the major effectors of mucosal immunity, are decreased both before and after exercise during major sports competition. It is possible that these results relate more to the effects of psychological stress than to the effects of exercise.

Salivary IgA concentration, espressed as μg IgA per mg protein, decreased significantly (p < 0.01) after each exercise session during both training and competition (Figure 2). The largest pre- to post-exercise decreases in IgA were observed after the two most difficult matches during competition (Comp 1 and Comp 3), as judged independently by the coach and manageress. Moreover, IgA concentration declined progressively over the

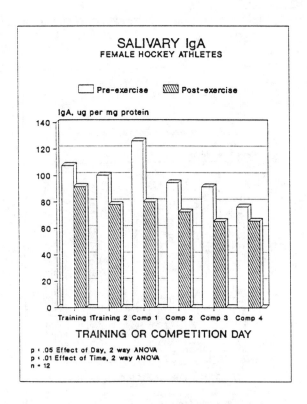

Figure 2. Salivary IgA concentration (μg/mg salivary protein) in female hockey athletes at the same times as in Figure 1. IgA levels decreased significantly (p < 0.01, 2-way ANOVA) after each exercise session during both training and competition. The exercise-induced decreases in IgA levels were largest after the most difficult competition matches (Comp 1 and 3). Resting IgA levels declined progressively over the five days of competition (p < 0.05, Neuman-Keuls post-hoc analysis for Comp 4 v's Comp 1).

five days of competitition; this trend was apparent for both pre- and post-exercise values, although of a larger magnitude for the pre-exercise values. These data suggest that the suppressive effects of daily intense exercise, at least during competition, may be cumulative over time.

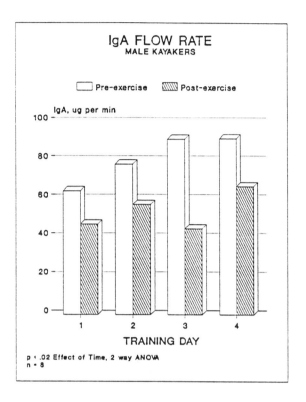

Figure 3. Salivary IgA flow rate (μg/min) for male kayakers before and after four training sessions over a one month period. IgA flow rates decreased after all sessions ($p < 0.02$, 2-way ANOVA). The largest decrease was observed after session 3, which occurred at the end of an especially intense week of training

STUDY 2 KAYAK STUDY

IgA flow rate, espressed as μg IgA per min, decreased markedly after all four training sessions ($p < .02$, Figure 3). IgA flow rates decreased to a similar extent (27%) after three sessions (1, 2, and 4); the largest decrease (51%) was noted after session 3, which was at the end of an especially intense week of training. Both resting and post--exercise IgA concentrations (μg per ml saliva) were also lowest on this day compared to other days (data not shown). The exercise-induced decreases in IgA flow rate were due mainly to a lower salivary flow rate, presumably due to dehydration. These data suggest that, although the concentration of IgA may not always change, the total amount of IgA available on the oral mucosal surface is reduced following intense exercise. In addition, there appears to be a cumulative effect of daily intense training on the resting IgA concentration and on the magnitude of exercise-induced decreases in IgA flow rate.

STUDY 3 SQUASH STUDY

Five of the 14 (36%) squash athletes became ill with URI during the ten week study period; this rate of illness agrees with anecdotal statements from athletes as well as published data.[3] There were a total of seven episodes of illness (one subject was ill on three occasions), all of which were classified as viral URI by the team physician; all episodes were rated as mild to moderate by athletes and the physician. No other illnesses were reported during this period.

For analysis the data were categorized into three groups: data from athletes who did not exhibit illness (Never Ill); the five athletes who became ill, but with saliva samples

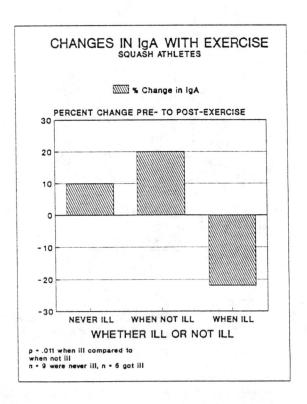

Figure 4. Percent changes in IgA concentration from pre- to post-exercise in squash athletes during weekly training. Data are grouped according to whether the athletes were developing illness at the time of sampling (see text for details). IgA concentration decreased after exercise in both groups of athletes who were not developing illness. IgA concentration decreased after exercise in the group of five athletes who became ill within two days after saliva sampling. (Neuman-Keuls post-hoc analysis revealed a significant difference between groups When Not Ill and When Ill.)

obtained when they were not ill (When Not Ill); and the five athletes who became ill, but with samples obtained within two days prior to their exhibiting illness (When Ill).

Data in Figure 4 show the percent differences between pre- and post-exercise IgA concentration (μg per ml saliva) in the three groups. IgA concentration increased 10 to 20% during exercise in both groups of athletes when they were not developing illness. In contrast, IgA concentration decreased 22% (p = .011, one way ANOVA on the pre- to post-exercise differences) in athletes who exhibited URI within two days after the saliva samples were obtained.

Chi square analysis of the frequency of illness related to changes in IgA levels indicated a highly significant distribution (p < .01, Table 1). Six of the seven episodes of URI were preceeded by decreases in IgA concentration (μg per ml) following exercise. To our knowledge, these are the first data showing a temporal relationship beween decreases in IgA concentration following exercise and subsequent URI.

It is unclear why an exercise-induced decrease in IgA levels preceeded illness in these athletes. It is possible that the athletes were already ill at the time of sampling and the exercise may have been more difficult than usual. It is also possible that some other factor, such as stress, influenced both IgA levels and resistance to infection. Clearly not all decreases in IgA were associated with illness; for example, IgA decreased following exercise on 27% of occasions when athletes were

Table 1. Changes in IgA with exercise - χ^2 analysis.

	Decreased IgA		No Decrease IgA	
	Obs.	(Exp.)	Obs.	(Exp.)
Never Ill	22	(20.0)	35	(36.9)
Got Ill, When Not Ill	5	(10.5)	25	(19.5)
Got Ill, When Ill	6	(2.5)	1	(4.5)

Data are presented as number of observations (94 total) for 14 athletes over a 10 week period. Observations were classified as to whether IgA concentration decreased or did not decrease (no change or increase in IgA) for each of the 3 groups (see text for details). χ^2 analysis revealed a highly significant ($\chi^2 = 12.58$, p < 0.01) distribution of data. Six of the seven episodes of illness were preceded within 2 days by a decrease in IgA following exercise.

not developing illness. These data may indicate an increased susceptibility to illness when IgA levels decrease during exercise; subsequent development of illness may then require other factors such as exposure to a specific microorganism or impairment of other aspects of immune function. These data were obtained on a relatively small sample group over a short period of time, and we are currently attempting to replicate these findings in a larger group of athletes over a longer period of time.

V. SUMMARY AND CONCLUSIONS

1.   Resting salivary IgA and IgM concentrations (μg per ml saliva) were lower during major sports competition compared to training.

2.   IgA concentration (μg per mg salivary protein) decreased immediately after exercise during both training and competition. The largest decreases occurred after the most intense competitive matches. Both resting and post-exercise IgA concentrations declined progressively over five days of major competition.

3.   IgA flow rate (μg per min) decreased after regular training sessions. The largest decrease was observed during a session at the end of an especially intense week of training. Both resting and post-exercise IgA concentration (μg per ml) were also lowest on this day compared to other training days.

4.   A temporal relationship was observed between decreases in IgA concentration (μg per ml) following exercise and appearance of upper respiratory illness.

These data suggest that IgA concentration, the amount of IgA relative to other proteins, and the total amount of IgA on the oral mucosal surfaces are all decreased during intense endurance exercise. These changes in mucosal immunoglobulin levels occurring during sports training and competition may be related to an increased incidence of upper respiratory illness in elite athletes. Stress, either psychological or physical or both, appears to influence immunoglobulin levels as well as the magnitude of exercise-induced changes.

VI. ACKNOWLEDGEMENTS

We gratefully acknowledge the enthusiastic cooperation of the coaches and team members of the following groups: The Queensland Senior Women's Hockey Team, the Australian Canoe Federation Kayak Unit, and the Australian Institute of Sport Squash Unit. This work was supported by a grant from the Australian Sports Commission.

VII. REFERENCES

1.   Douglas, D.J. and Hanson, P.G., Upper respiratory infections in the conditioned athlete, *Med.Sci.Sports Exerc.*, 10, 55, 1978.
2.   Tomasi, T.B., Trudeau, F.B., Czerwinski, D. and Erredge, S., Immune parameters in athletes before and after strenuous exercise, *J.Clin.Immunol.*, 2, 173, 1982.

3.   Peters, E.M. and Bateman, E.D., Ultramarathon running and upper respiratory tract infections: An epidemiological survey, *Sth.Afr.Med.J.*, 64, 582, 1983.

4.   Nieman, D.C., Johanssen, L.M. and Lee, J.W., Infectious episodes in runners before and after a road race, *J.Sports Med.Physical Fitness*, 29, 289, 1989.

5.   Mackinnon, L.T., Chick, T.W., van As, A. and Tomasi, T.B., The effect of severe prolonged exercise on the immune response, *Abstracts,Sixth International Congress of Immunology*, 56, 1986.(Abstract)

6.   Mackinnon, L.T., Chick, T.W., van As, A. and Tomasini, T.B., Decreased secretory immunoglobulins following intense prolonged exercise, *Sports Training Med.Rehab.*, 1, 1, 1989.

7.   Mackinnon, L.T., Ginn, E. and Seymour, G., Comparison of the effects of exercise during training and competition on secretory IgA levels, *Med.Sci.Sports Exerc.*, 22, S125, 1990.

8.   Muns, G., Liesen, H., Riedel, H. and Bergmann, K-C., Influence of long-distance running on IgA in nasal secretion and saliva, *Deutsche Zeitschrift fur Sportmedizin*, 40, 63, 1989.

9.   Tharp, G.D. and Barnes, M.W., Reduction of saliva immunoglobulin levels by swim training, *Eur.J.Appl.Physiol.*, 60, 61, 1990.

10.   Jemmott, J.B., Borysenko, M., Chapman, R. and et al., , Academic stress, power motivation, and decrease in secretion rate of salivary secretory immunoglobin A, *Lancet*, 1, 1400, 1983.

11.   Bird, P.S. and Seymour, G.J., Production of monoclonal antibodies that recognize specific and cross-reactive antigens of Fusobacterium nucleatum, *Infect.Immun.*, 55, 571, 1987.

V. Impact of Psychoimmunology in Clinical Medicine

ENDOGENOUS OPIATES, NATURAL KILLER CELLS AND PSYCHOSOCIAL FACTORS IN EARLY BREAST CANCER PATIENTS

Maryanne O'Donnell.

Department of Psychiatry, Prince of Wales Hospital, High Street, Randwick. NSW. 2031. Australia

I. ABSTRACT

The inability to express emotion has been consistently reported in psychosocial studies of cancer patients. Furthermore, expression of negative affect has been correlated with better survival in cancer patients. Speculation about the possible mediators of such effects has implicated central nervous system (CNS) regulation of the immune system but few studies have investigated possible pathways. This study of 53 patients with early stage breast cancer, investigated relationships between psychosocial factors, natural killer cell activity (NKCA), endogenous opioid levels and the patient's nodal status.

Patients who were nodes positive showed higher scores on the Courtauld Emotional Control suppression of anger subscale, thereby extending previous findings by implicating suppression of anger in the progression of neoplastic disease. Significant correlations between poor adjustment and NKCA indicate that expression of negative affect may be prognostically favourable and a significant inverse correlation between NKCA and β-endorphin levels suggests pathways that may mediate the effects of stress on NKCA.

II. INTRODUCTION

While it is important to acknowledge that the major aetiological factors in all cancers are undoubtedly physical (genetic factors, exposure to carcinogens etc.), and the major determinants of outcome are the biological characteristics of the tumour, there is growing body of evidence indicating that psychological factors may also influence the course of cancer.

This area of psychosocial oncology has been stimulated by findings in the burgeoning field of psychoneuroimmunology which is now providing compelling evidence that the CNS and the immune system can interact, and that ways of coping with stress and distress affect immune functioning.[1] Intensive biomedical research in oncology since the Second World War has been relatively unsuccessful in curbing the escalating incidence of cancer.[2] This failure has resulted in researchers following a more 'inclusive' model of health and illness, the biopsychosocial model, which asserts that disease may be usefully analysed at several different levels.

For centuries physicians have suggested that emotional expression may be involved in cancer onset and progression. Gross,[3] in a recent article, surveyed 18 studies which directly relate emotional expression to cancer onset and progression. The main findings suggest that women who express negative affect and anxiety have a better prognosis.[4,5] These seemingly paradoxical findings describe patients who may be hostile, anxious, assertive and whose management is often difficult compared to passive, compliant, accepting, perhaps easier to manage patients. Studies suggest that this expression of negative emotion is particularly relevant at the time of diagnosis and operation. Levy *et al*,[6] in a study on a cohort of breast cancer patients, found that women who were more distressed and maladjusted at the time of operation had a better prognosis. Also, Dean and Surtees[7] study found that patients who were regarded as having enough symptoms to fulfill the criteria for a psychiatric illness (according to the RDC & the GHQ) *before* operation were *less* likely to have a recurrence during follow-up whereas patients who had persistent symptoms at 3 months after operation had a poorer prognosis, so that high scorers on the GHQ did worse. The expression of distress at the time of diagnosis or operation may be an adaptive response (perhaps analogous to a normal grief response) whereas chronic distress may have deleterious effects.[3]

In accord with these findings that cancer patients who express emotion have a better prognosis are findings reporting an inability to express emotion in cancer patients. In particular, a lifelong pattern of suppression of anger has been shown.[8,9] Earlier studies used non-standardised interviews to assess suppression or anger but more recently Watson and Greer have developed the Courtauld Emotional Control Scale, a patient-rated scale with three subscales measuring suppression of anxiety, anger and depression.[10] Using this scale, they demonstrated that breast cancer patients had significantly higher scores on the suppression of anger scale than patients with benign breast disease. Converging findings in this area have led to the notion of a type 'C' or cancer prone individual who is characterised as cooperative, and unassertive and who suppresses negative emotion, particularly anger. Temoshok *et al*[11] found this personality construct to be significantly correlated with tumour thickness, a prognostic indicator in malignant melanoma patients.

If emotional expression is important in cancer patients, what are the likely mediators of such an effect?

For pychoimmunology to be relevant to cancer research, it is essential that tumours are able to elicit an immune response. Over the past few years, specific immunological reactions have been demonstrated in patients with tumours of all types although some classes of tumours are more weakly antigenic than others.[12] The cytotoxic activity of Natural Killer Cells (NKC) has cells has attracted considerable attention. These lymphocytes are of uncertain lineage but are clearly controlkd by T cells and are known as 'stress' lymphocytes. Several studies have demonstrated decreased NKCA in association with depression, loneliness and poor coping ability.[13,14] Cytokines, like interferon-γ, are known to stimulate their activity. NK cells are capable of spontaneous cytotoxic activity against a wide range of tumours and, because they require no prior sensitisation to their targets and are capable of mounting a rapid response, it has been suggested that they provide the first line of defence against the emergence of tumours or their metastases.[15] Higher levels of NKCA have been reported in breast cancer patients whose axillary lymph nodes were not invaded compared with patients with axillary spread of disease pointing to a role for NKCA in the prevention of metastases.[6]

The discovery of receptor sites on the surface of immune cells for catecholamines, steroid hormones and opiate peptides suggest specific neuroendocrine pathways which may directly influence the functioning of immune cells.[16] The neuropeptides, β-endorphin and Met-Enkephalin are released in response to stress and have both immunoenhancing and immunoinhibitory effects on NKCA.[17] In acute stress, these neuropeptides seem to enhance NKCA whereas chronic stress appears to reduce NKCA.

Although there has been considerable speculation about how these mechanisms may be relevant in oncogenesis, only a few studies have investigated links between psychological factors and the immune system in cancer patients. Pettingale et al,[18] in a study of women with breast cancer and control subjects with benign breast disease, found that increased serum IgA levels were correlated with life long suppression of anger. Levy et al[6] demonstrated increased NKCA in breast cancer patients rated as poorly adjusted on the Derogatis Global Adjustment to Illness Scale (GAIS) compared to their well adjusted counterparts.

In an attempt to identify possible biological mediators of behavioural factors the present study invatigated relationships between psychological factors, endogenous opioids, measures of immunoreactivity and survival in a group of breast cancer patients.

III. METHOD

Fifty three patients attending the Radiotherapy Clinic at the Prince of Wales HospitaL aged less than 65 yrs, with early stage disease ($T_{0,1,2}$; $N_{0,1}$; M_0), agreed to participate in the study. All were due to undergo radiotherapy to the chest wall 4-6 weeks developing surgery. Patients were interviewed at the time they presented for radiotherapy planning. They were asked about their attitudes to their diagnosis and rated on the GAIS by two independent raters. Patients were then given five standardised psychological tests measuring state and trait anxiety (STAI), depression (BDI), loneliness (UCLA), locus of control (LCB) and emotional control (CECS). These tests were returned by patients within two days or the initial interview, at which point blood was collected to measure NKCA, γ-interferon, β-endorphin, and Met-Enkephalin levels. All blood samples were collected between 0700h-0900h to control for circadian rhythmicity.

Although our ultimate objective is to determine correlations between behavioural factors and recurrence of disease, because no data is yet available on the 5 year survival rates of these patients, histological node status was used as a *correlate* of survival as it is considered a major prognostic indicator in early stage breast cancer.[19]

IV. RESULTS

Of the 53 patients involved, 26 patients had mastectomies and 27 lumpectomies. There were no signiffcant correlations between the type of operation or the menopausal status of the patients and any of the psychosocial variables tested. Similarly, there was no significant correlation between age and any of the psychological tests, ratings of adjustment and levels of NKCA or endogenous opioids. γ-interferon levels were insignificant in all patients and will not be discussed further. Twenty seven patients were classified as nodes negative. Of the 26 patients classifed as positive, 1-17 nodes were invaded by disease (Mean=1.4). Age was signifcantly associated with nodal status (r=0.3, p=.01).

There was a significant inverse relationship between NKCA and β-endorphin (r=-.30, p=.03). This negative correlation was only significant in the group of patients who were treated with mastectomy rather than lumpectomy. Partialling out the effects of psychosocial variables like anxiety, depression and emotional control did not diminish this relationship. In the present study we were unable to demonstrate increased NKCA in patients whose axillary nodes were not invaded by disease (r=22, p=.08).

Table 1.   Spearman correlations between adjustment to illness and biological variables (n=43)

	GAIS Score	
	Rater 1	Rater 2
NATURAL KILLER CELL ACTIVITY	-.25*	-.26
β-ENDORPHIN	-.3	.17
MET-ENKEPHALIN	.05	.14

* p=.05

As can be seen from Table 1, patients rated lower on the GAIS (ie. those patients rated as 'less well adjusted'), by both raters, had significantly higher kvels of NKCA. Although 53 patients entered the study there is only complete data available on 43 patients due to some technical difficulties in testing some or the biological assays.

As can be seen from Table 2, patients rated as 'poorly adjusted' had significantly higher scores on psychological tests measuring the negative affects of depression, loneliness, anxiety and external locus of control.

Suppression of emotion scores were not associated with ratings of adjustment but were significantly correlated with nodal status. Patients who were nodes positive had significantly higher scores on the suppression of anger subscale of the emotional control scale. One way analysis of variance revealed that the mean suppression of anger scores for the nodes positive group was significantly higher than for the nodes negative group (F=5.09, df=1,49, p=0.03).

There was a trend, not reaching significance, for total suppression of emotion scores to be higher for the nodes positive group. Neither the suppression of anxiety or depression subscales scores were significantly higher in the nodes positive group. Step wise multiple regression was undertaken to determine the variables which best predicted nodal status. Age was significantly associated with nodal status and accounted for 14% of the variance (p = .006). Suppression of anger scores accounted for a further 11% of the variance in nodal status (p = .001).

Table 2. Spearman correlations between psychological tests and adjustment (n = 49-52)

	GAIS Score	
	Rater 1	Rater 2
DEPRESSION (BDI)	-.34**	-.42***
LONELINESS (UCLA)	-.23*	.23*
ANXIETY (STAI)		
-STATE	-.49***	-.20
-TRAIT	-.40**	-.31*
LOCUS OF CONTROL (LCB)	-.57***	-.15

* p = .05, ** p < .01, *** p < .001

V. DISCUSSION

We have partially replicated findings of Levy et al[6] by demonstrating significant correlations between NKCA and ratings of poorer adjustment. The psychohgical profiles of patients rated as poorly adjusted indicate that these patients express negative affect lending support to previous findings.[4-7] It will be important to examine follow up data to distinguish between patients expressing negative affect at the time of radiotherapy planning and those who persistently express negative affect to determine different effects on survival.

We have been unable to replicate Levy et al[6] findings of higher NKCA in patients with no nodes involved. This may indicate that NKCA plays no role in the prevention or metastases, or reflect differences between the two studies. In the current study, NKCA was measured at 4-6 weeks postoperatively whereas Levy et al[6] measured NKCA one week following surgery.

The finding of a significant inverse *in vivo* correlation between NKCA and β-endorphin in the mastectomy but not lumpectomy patients suggests an immunosuppressive relationship in this group. Possibly mastectomy produces more sustained arousal then lumpectomy in which case this finding points to a role for arousal in the mediation of this effect. This inverse relationship could be influenced by psychosocial factors or be a post operative physiological response. The previous linking of NKCA with adjustment indicates the need for further clarification of the relationship between the endorphins and NKCA.

Our findings corroborate the results of previous studies[8,9,11] which examined the rolek of suppression of anger in cancer onset and progression. Using the suppression of anger subscale, administered pre-operatively, Pettingale *et al*[20] were able to discrimmate between patients with benign breast tumours and those with cancer. Our findings, in diagnosed patients, suggest that suppression of anger may be implicated in the progression of neoplastic disease. We have been unablek to demonstrate any direct link between suppression of anger and NKCA leaving it unclear whether these immune cells are involved in the mediation of the processes underlying suppression of emotion and progression of disease.

Our results indicate that the role of expression of emotion in cancer patients is worthy of further study and suggest that attempts to maximise management of malignancy may require better understanding of personality factors and coping skills. This may have implications for management of cancer patients by ensuring that there is adequate opportunity for them to express their feelings on learning their diagnoses and that the expression of negative affect is not inhibited. Before long term strategies could be considered however, we need further clarification of what exactly is being measured in suppression of emotion and its physiological response. As yet, the physiology of emotion is poorly understood. Although we have examined several biological meaures, it is becoming increasingly clear that the likely mediating mechanisms involve complex cascades of humoral substances which are governed by feedback mechanisms and regulatory circuits, the investigation of which is necessary to the clarification of the role that suppression of emotion plays in cancer onset and progression.

VI. ACKNOWLEDGEMENTS

Dr. Maryanne O'Donnell was supported by a Research Fellowship from the N.S.W. Institute of Psychiatry. Thanks are expressed to Associate Professor N. McConaghy, Professor J. Dwyer and Dr. N. Wilton for the supervision of this project, the Radiotherapy Department for their co-operation, and to Dr. P. Ward and Dr. A. Blaszczynski for assistance with the statistics.

VII. REFERENCES

1.   Calabrese, J.R., Kling, M.A. and Gold, P.W., Alterations in immunocompetence during stress, bereavement and depression: Focus on neuroendocrine regulation, *Am.J.Psychiatr.*, 144, 1123, 1987.

2.   Bailar, J.C.I and Smith, E.M., Progress against Cancer, *New Eng.J.Med.*, 314, 1226, 1986.

3.   Gross, J., Emotional expression in cancer onset and progression, *Soc.Sci.Med.*, 28, 1239, 1989.

4.   Derogatis, L.R., Abeloff, M.D. and Melisaratos, N., Psychological coping mechanisms and survival time in metastatic breast cancer, *J.A.M.A.*, 242, 1504,

1979.

5. Jensen, M.R., Psychobiological factors predicting the course of breast cancer, *J.Personality*, 55, 317, 1987.

6. Levy, S.M., Herberman, R.B., Maluish, A.M., Schlien, B. and Lippman, M., Prognostic risk factors in primary breast cancer by behavioural and immunological parameters, *Hlth.Psych.*, 4, 99, 1985.

7. Dean, C. and Surtees, P.G., Do psychological factors predict survival in breast cancer ? *J.Psychosom.Res.*, 33, 561, 1989.

8. Morris, T., Greer, S., Pettingale, K.W. and Watson, M., Patterns of expression of anger and their psychological correlates in women with breast cancer, *J.Psychosom.Res.*, 28, 117, 1984.

9. Kissen, D.M., Personality characteristics in males conducive to lung cancer patients, *Br.J.med.Psych.*, 36, 27, 1963.

10. Watson, M. and Greer, S., Development of a questionnaire measure of emotional control, *J.Psychosom.Res.*, 27, 299, 1983.

11. Temoshok, L., Heller, B.W., Sagebiel, R.W., Blois, M.S., Sweet, D.M., DiClemente, R.J. and Gold, M.L., The relationship of psychosocial factors to prognostic indicators in cutaneous malignant melanoma, *J.Psychosom.Res.*, 29, 139, 1985.

12. Pettingale, K.W., Towards a psychobiological model of cancer: Biological considerations, *Soc.Sci.Med.*, 20, 779, 1985.

13. Locke, S.E., Kraus, L., Leserman, J., Hurst, M.W., Heisal, S. and Williams, R.M., Life change stress, psychiatric symptoms, and natural killer cell activity, *Psychosom.Med.*, 46, 441, 1991.

14. Kiecolt-Glaser, J.K. and Glaser, R., Psychological influences on immunity, *Psychosomatics*, 27, 621, 1986.

15. Herberman, R.B., Natural killer cells, *Ann.Rev.Med.*, 37, 347, 1986.

16. Tecoma, E.S. and Huey, L.Y., Psychic distress and the immune response, *Life Sci.*, 36, 1799, 1985.

17. Greenberg, A.H., Dyck, D.G. and Sandler, L.S., Opponent processes, neurohormones and natural resistance, in *Impact of Psychoendocrine Systems in Cancer and Immunity*, Fox, B.H. and Newberry, B.H., Eds., C.J. Hogrefe, Inc., New York, 1984.

18. Pettingale, K.W., Greer, S. and Tee, D.E.H., Serum IgA and emotional expression in breast cancer patients, *J.Psychosom.Res.*, 21, 395, 1977.

19. Henderson, I.C. and Canellos, G.P., Cancer of the breast, The past decade, *New Eng.J.Med.*, 302, 17, 1980.

20. Pettingale, K.W., Watson, M. and Greer, S., The validity of emotional control as a trait in breast cancer patients, *J.Psychosoc.Oncology*, 2, 21, 1985.

THE EFFECT OF A MULTIMODAL STRESS MANAGEMENT PROGRAM ON IMMUNE AND PSYCHOLOGICAL FUNCTIONS

A. Blenkhorn, D. Silove[a], C. Magarey, S. Krillis and H. Colinet

Department Surgery, St. George Hospital,
and [a]Department of Psychiatry, Liverpool Hospital. NSW Australia.

I. ABSTRACT

This investigation was a pilot study, examining the effects of a multimodal stress management program on psychological and immune functions in a sample of subjects most of whom were the relatives and friends of cancer patients. Baseline psychological and immunological results revealed that the subjects were significantly distressed and immuno-suppressed, and post-intervention results demonstrated that there were significant improvements in psychological well-being, and that these improvements were maintained for the small number of subjects completing six week follow up.

However, the immunological effects of the intervention were less clear-cut, with the *in vivo* Delayed Hypersensitivity Skin Tests showing improvements in the number of positive responses for the group as a whole, while the total induration score only showed significant improvement in a small group of subjects. The results for the Phytohaemaglutinin (PHA) stimulation of lymphocytes assay revealed that there was a significant decline in *in vitro* lymphocyte responsiveness for one concentration of PHA.

II. INTRODUCTION

A common theme developing in the psychosomatic literature is that the immune system is affected by psychological influences and that these changes in immune function may, in turn, affect the diseases process.[1,2]

In the last five years there have been a number of studies using psychological interventions aimed at enhancing immune functions. Peavey *et al*[3] studied the effects of biofeedback-assisted relaxation (BAR) on phagocytic activity in a group of volunteers. Initially they entered 41 subjects into the study. Sixteen of these subjects were found to have significantly high stress scores and low immunity compared to the other 25 subjects. These 16 subjects were randomly allocated into control and intervention (BAR) groups. The intervention group's phagocytic activity significantly increased compared to their own pre-intervention levels and the control group. There was also a significant reduction in anxiety and tension in the intervention group. Smith *et al*[4] investigated whether an experienced meditator could alter her delayed hypersensitivity skin test (DHST) reaction and lymphocyte stimulation response to the Varicella Zoster viral antigen. The subject had three baseline, three intervention, and three follow up tests at weekly intervals. The results showed that compared to baseline and follow up scores, during the "specific" intervention periods, the subject was able to decrease significantly both her skin test response, and the blastogenic response of her lymphocytes. Similarly, Rider *et al*[5], were able to show that with the use of music-assisted mental imagery, subjects were able to alter significantly peripheral neutrophil and lymphocyte counts after a six week training period.

Other researchers have examined the effects of relaxation and social support on immune function. Kiecolt-Glaser *et al*[6] randomly allocated 45 healthy geriatric subjects to three groups, subjects in the relaxation and social support groups received sessions lasting 45 minutes, three times a week for a month, while the control group did not receive any intervention. Natural Killer cell activity increased significantly in the relaxation group, with no comparable changes in the other two groups. There was also a significant decrease in antibody titres to the Herpes Simplex Virus and self rated distress scores only in the relaxation group. However, these improvements in psychological and immune function did not persist at follow up, one month later. This study showed that relaxation may be an important factor in improving some immune functions but that an increase in social contact does not, on its own, achieve the same effects. Kiecolt-Glaser *et al*[7] conducted another intervention study, this time with medical students, to assess the benefits of relaxation in alleviating the psychological distress and immune suppression seen in students undertaking examinations. Thirty four subjects were randomly allocated to relaxation and control groups and completed psychological questionnaires and immune tests one month prior to, and on the second day of examinations. Relaxation sessions ran for 35-45 minutes and included standard 'deepening' exercises, self hypnosis, autogenic training, and various imagery exercises. Immunologically, there were decreases in the percentages of T helper cells, and the T helper/T suppressor ratio. The frequency of relaxation practice predicted the percentage of T helper cells after the intervention, with a high frequency of practice being associated with higher percentages of T helper cells. Kiecolt-Glaser *et al*[7] suggested that their two intervention studies "provide further evidence that relaxation may be able to enhance at least some components of cellular immunity and, thus, perhaps ultimately might be useful in influencing the incidence and course of disease".

The above studies together provide preliminary evidence that immune function can be altered by the practice of relaxation, meditation, and visual imagery. However, the body of existing data is small and much further work is required to confirm these findings. Also, in most studies, subjects (such as medical students) have been used which do not reflect the reality of clinical practice. For these reasons, subjects were selected on the basis that they were assumed to be distressed, clinically relevant and in need. Most of the subjects were the friends and relatives of cancer patients, a group of subjects that has been shown to be highly distressed and in need of help.[8] Furthermore caregivers of the chronically ill such as Alzheimer's sufferers, have been shown to be immunologically suppressed[9], and recently a report has shown similar levels of distress in family caregivers of Alzheimer's disease patients and caregivers of cancer patients.[10]

The aims of this study were therefore to evaluate the effects of a multimodal stress reduction program on alleviating psychological distress and enhancing immune functions. It was hypothesised that study subjects, most of whom would be the friends and relatives of cancer patients, would be psychologically distressed, that the intervention would reduce this psychological distress and improve *in vivo* and *in vitro* cell mediated immunity.

III. MATERIALS AND METHODS

Subjects were recruited into the study through an article published in the local newspaper and through the cancer clinic at St. George Hospital, a principal teaching Hospital of The University of New South Wales, Australia. Subjects were assembled for an introductory meeting and given a detailed description of the intervention and research design before they were invited to consent to participate. They were then randomly allocated into one of two groups, an intervention group which would enter the stress management program immediately, and a control group which would wait during this period and then participate in the next intervention group. Subjects were randomly allocated in a manner which allowed family members and friends to remain together with the rest of each family/friend unit accompanying the index subject into the same group.

Each group meeting extended for 2 hours on successive Wednesday evenings for six weeks. At each meeting subjects practiced 20 minutes of deep muscle relaxation, participated in general discussions and sharing of experiences concerned with practising meditation. A short talk was then given illustrating pertinent experiences and strategies for dealing with cancer, eg methods for supporting cancer patients, issues relating to death and dying and approaches to self-care. Subjects then formed smaller groups convened by experienced councillors who lead discussions, encouraging the sharing of experiences and strategies in dealing with cancer distress. Finally, participants were instructed in the practice of meditation, and were encouraged to practice meditation each day so that it would eventually become an integral part of their daily routine. Meditation techniques were taught by an experienced meditator, who has practised meditation for a number of years. Subjects were led through a series of exercises which relax the mind and body e.g. visualising themselves in a peaceful environment or focusing their attention on their breathing.

TIMING AND TYPE OF TESTS

Subjects filled out a proforma which included a number of psychological questionnaires, demographic data and questions concerning behaviours known to effect immune function as described below. The investigators then drew a 20 ml blood sample and administered a delayed hypersensitivity skin test. These tests were repeated after six weeks, and were possible, a further six weeks later. The immune tests were conducted at the same time of day to control for possible diurnal variations in immune function.[11] Subjects were asked to report on risk factors known to affect immune function,[11] namely, any recent illness, recent changes in sleeping habits, the number of alcoholic drinks per week, the number of cigarettes smoked per day, any recent changes in weight, and medication use.

PSYCHOLOGICAL QUESTIONNAIRES

The General Health Questionnaire (30 Item) (GHQ) is a general screening measure for non-psychotic psychiatric illness, with extensive normative information on overseas and Australian communities.[12,13] It consists of a series of questions about current symptoms, abnormal feelings and thoughts, and aspects of observable behaviour.[13] The GHQ was scored according to the method of Goodchild and Duncan-Jones.[12] Profile of Mood States (POMS) is an extensive measure of emotional state, which quantifies symptoms such as depression, tension, and anxiety in moderately disturbed groups. Its utility in longitudinal psychotherapy studies is well documented.[14]

IMMUNOLOGICAL TESTS

For measures of *in vitro* immune function, phytohaemaglutinnin (PHA) mitogen stimulation of lymphocytes was employed. This test has been well established as a general measure of cell mediated immunity in numerous studies.[15-17] Subjects peripheral blood was drawn into syringes containing preservative-free heparin. Mononuclear cells were separated by the Ficoll separation method[18] and cryopreserved according to Golub.[19] The PHA mitogen stimulation of lymphocytes was carried out using standard techniques.[18] Triplicate 100 μl aliquotes of both the cell suspension and the various concentrations of PHA/RPMI were placed in a sterile 96 flat well microtitre plates. The final cell concentration was 1×10^6 cells/ml. The cells were incubated in 5% CO_2 at 37°C for 72 hours. The cells were then pulsed with 50 μl of tritiated thymidine (0.85 μCi per well) for 16 hours, and then harvested onto glass fibre filters (Cambridge Technology) using a semi automated cell harvester (PHD Cell Harvester, Cambridge Technology Inc.). Beta emissions were counted on a Tri-Carb 4000 Series Liquid Scintillation System Beta Counter for 1 minute. Results were recorded in disintegrations per minute (DPM) and the mean of the triplicate samples calculated. The stimulation of mononuclear cells was calculated by subtracting the control sample (no PHA) from the stimulated samples (with PHA) and log10 transformed. The samples taken at different times for each subject were tested on the same plate at the same time to reduce the amount of experimental variation that is seen in this assay on a day to day basis.

The Multitest C.M.I. from Institut Merieux France was used to evaluate Delayed Hypersensitivity in subjects. In evaluating the skin test scores we followed the same procedure as Kniker *et al*[20], using both the number of positive responses, and the total induration score to quantify the results.

STATISTICAL ANALYSIS

Data were coded and entered into an IBM compatible computer. The statistical analyses were conducted using the Statistics Package for Social Sciences (SPSS) program. In all of the hypotheses tested, the 0.05 level of probability was utilized. Due to the complex nature of the research design four different statistical tests were carried out to determine the significance of changes in psychological and immune function.

Within Subjects Design. As will be seen below, the Case-Control comparison included a reduced sample size because of the complex design outlined in Figure 1. For this reason it was judged to be valuable to conduct exploratory univariate analyses on all the subjects completing the intervention to maximise statistical power. Two-tailed paired t-tests were conducted to compare the pre and post intervention, and the pre and post control period scores to assess changes over the six week periods.

Case-Control Design. The case-control analyses are based on the random allocation design. The statistical analysis employed was a 2 X 2 mutivariate analysis of variance (MANOVA).

Repeated Measures Design 1: (Control Group 'Cross Over' to Intervention Group.). The repeated measures design 1 analysis was conducted on the results from subjects who completed all three tests (PRETEST 1, PRETEST 2, POSTTEST). These subjects were

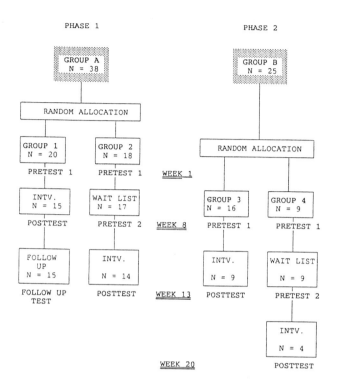

Figure 1. Research design illustrating random allocation, number of subjects tested (N), time of tests and time of entry into the study. (Intv. = Intervention)

initially randomly allocated into the 6 week waiting list control group, and then "crossed over" to complete the intervention. This design allows the detection of changes over the waiting period (PRETEST 1 versus PRETEST 2) and, taking the average of the two pre intervention scores gives a more accurate estimate of baseline scores to compare with the post intervention score. These analyses were performed using the repeated measures MANOVA.

Repeated Measures Design 2: (Intervention Plus Six Week Follow Up Tests). To determine if there were any carry over effects in the 6 weeks following the intervention, the repeated measures design 2 was conducted on subjects who completed the three tests, PRETEST 1, POSTTEST and FOLLOW UP TESTS. These analyses were performed using the repeated measures MANOVA.

IV. RESULTS

The study involved two intervention groups treated consecutively, and two waiting list control groups. As shown in Figure 1, at the first meeting (Phase 1, Week 1) 38 consenting subjects (Group A) were randomly allocated to either a treatment group (Group 1), or a wait list control group (Group 2). After the six weeks intervention period (Phase 2, Week 8), another 25 subjects (Group B) entered the study and were randomly allocated to either the treatment group (Group 3) or the wait list control group (Group 4). Groups 2 and 3 then completed the 6 week intervention program together, while Group 4 waited. At the end of the six week period (Week 13) all groups completed tests including Group 1 which had six week follow up tests, and then Group 4 entered the intervention program, completing post intervention tests at week 20.

This gave a total of 63 subjects who volunteered to participate in the study. Because of time constraints, only Group 1 subjects completed follow up tests. (see Figure 1) Group 1 subjects were not given any further intervention program during the follow up period, but all reported continuing to practice meditation. The number of subjects completing tests (N) quoted in Figure 1, are based on subjects who completed the Delayed Hypersensitivity Skin Tests (DHST). The number of subjects included in the other analyses varies slightly, because some subjects completed questionnaires incorrectly, and in the case of the PHA immune tests, subjects in Group 4 were not tested due to research time constraints.

DEMOGRAPHIC DATA

Demographic data for the volunteers is presented in Table 1. Forty two subjects were the friends and relatives of patients with cancer, and 21 were people either suffering from stress related problems or who wanted to learn meditation and relaxation techniques. For the intervention and control groups Chi-square analysis indicated there were no significant demographic differences between the two groups, however there were more subjects in the intervention (N=36) than the control group (N=27). This difference between the number of

TABLE 1
DEMOGRAPHIC DATA FOR ALL SUBJECTS

NUMBER OF SUBJECTS		N = 63
AGE	mean 49 yrs	(range 16 - 77)
SEX	MALE 21	FEMALE 42
MARITAL STATUS	MARRIED	44
	DEFACTO	1
	SINGLE	10
	DIVORCED	2
	WIDOWED	6
EDUCATION	TERTIARY	21
	SECONDARY	42

subjects in the two groups was due to two reasons. First, the randomly allocated family/friend units were not of equal size, and secondly, some subjects who were allocated to the control group could not wait for six weeks to take part in the intervention, and were entered into the intervention group for ethical reasons.

All 63 subjects completed baseline tests. As shown in Figure 1, a maximum of 42 of the 63 subjects completed both Pretest 1 and Posttest intervention tests, and 26 of the 28 control subjects completed both Pretest 1 and Pretest 2 tests over the waiting period. The attrition in the number of subjects over the course of the study was due to a number of factors; a) some subjects dropped out; b) others had spouses who were receiving cancer treatment and the constraints they faced meant they could not find the time to complete the tests; c) one subject moved to another state; and d) some subjects completed questionnaires incorrectly.

SELF REPORT DATA

At baseline 37 of the 63 subjects reported taking medication, 16 reported sleep disturbances, 8 recent weight 1088, 13 smoking cigarettes and 11 consuming more than two alcoholic drinks per day. The percentage of subjects reporting these behaviours did not change significantly at post control period, post intervention and six week follow up reports.

SELF RATING PSYCHOLOGICAL SCALES

The General Health Questionnaire (GHQ). Using the scoring method of Goodchild and Duncan-Jones,[12] scores above 12 indicate that the subject is sufficiently symptomatic to

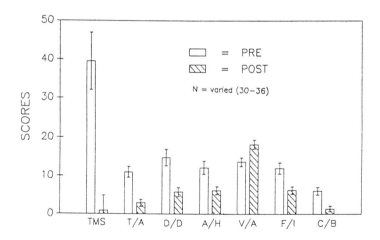

Figure 2. Profile of mood states. Mean ($\pm$ SE) PRE and POST scores for all subjects completing the intervention.

be considered in need of psychiatric help. The normal population would be expected to return scores of 7-8. For the 23 subjects completing pre and post intervention and the 22 subjects completing pre and post control period tests their respective mean (SD) scores were 14.3 (7.5) and 18.3 (7.5), which were well above the level for "caseness" indicating that, as a group, these subjects were substantially psychologically distressed.

The Profile of Mood States Questionnaire (POMS). The POMS results for the Within Subjects Design are represented in Figure 2 for the intervention group, and Figure 3 for the control group. Paired t-test comparisons of pre intervention (PRE 1) and post intervention (POST) scores showed a highly statistically significant improvement in psychological well-being as measured by the six dimensions and the TMS after the intervention (p < 0.001 for all dimensions and TMS), and no significant change for the control group. Note, the number of subjects completing the POMS varies for some of the dimensions and the TMS, which is due to subjects completing questionnaires incorrectly.

Group means and standard deviations for the Case-Control Design analysis are presented in Table 2. The MANOVA analysis revealed that over the six week period the intervention group scores changed significantly more than the control group for five of the six POMS dimensions and the TMS, with the most significant change being Depression/Dejection ($F[1,38] = 8.60$, $p < 0.005$) and Tension/Anxiety ($F[1,38] = 16.32$, $p < 0.0001$). For the other POMS dimensions the level of probability was less than 0.05, while the change for Confusion/Bewilderment approached significance ($p < 0.06$).

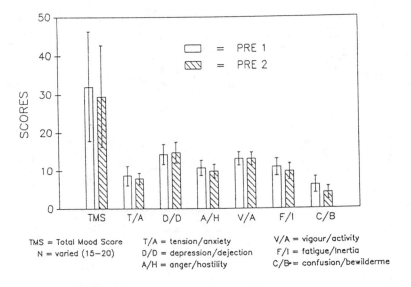

TMS = Total Mood Score   T/A = tension/anxiety   V/A = vigour/activity
N = varied (15–20)   D/D = depression/dejection   F/I = fatigue/inertia
                             A/H = anger/hostility   C/B = confusion/bewilderme

Figure 3. Profile of mood states. Mean (± SE) control group scores before (PRE 1) and after   (PRE 2) the 6 week waiting period.

TABLE 2. CASE-CONTROL DESIGN:PRE AND POST MEANS FOR THE
INTERVENTION AND CONTROL GROUPS   PROFILE OF MOOD STATES
(POMS) QUESTIONNAIRE.(Standard deviations in parenthesis)

	GROUP:	INTERVENTION N = (22-20)[a]	CONTROL N = (19-17)[a]
Total Mood Score	Pre	44.4*** (44.1)	31.6 (56.7)
	Post	1.1 (26.2)	30.3 (52.8)
Depression/Dejection	Pre	16.2 (13.4)	14.4 (15.0)
	Post	5.6** (7.7)	14.9 (15.6)
Anger/Hostility	Pre	12.0 (9.9)	10.6 (12.2)
	Post	5.3* (5.7)	10.1 (10.7)
Tension/Anxiety	Pre	12.3 (8.5)	8.8 (10.2)
	Post	2.7*** (5.8)	8.4 (8.7)
Vigour/Activity	Pre	13.7 (5.9)	13.6 (7.2)
	Post	17.7* (7.3)	13.7 (7.1)
Fatigue/Inertia	Pre	13.2 (8.8)	11.0 (9.0)
	Post	6.1* (5.8)	10.1 (8.7)
Confusion/Bewilderment	Pre	7.1 (5.9)	6.0 (8.6)
	Post	1.9 (4.4)	4.2 (6.8)

* p < 0.04, ** p < 0.005, *** p < 0.0001 N values
variation due to subjects completing questionnaires
incorrectly.

The POMS results for subjects completing the two pre intervention tests (PRE 1 and PRE 2) and post intervention tests (POST) are presented in Table 3. There was a significant difference between the average of the two pre intervention (PRE 1 and PRE 2) and the post intervention scores (POST) for Vigour/Activity, (p < 0.003) and Fatigue/Inertia, (p < 0.05). While there were trends for the other dimensions of the POMS scale, they were not statistically significant, most likely representing a Type 1 error due to the small number of subjects completing the tests (N = 7 to 12).

TABLE 3. REPEATED MEASURES DESIGN 1: MEAN PROFILE OF MOOD
STATES (POMS) SCORES FOR SUBJECTS COMPLETING PRE AND POST
CONTROL PERIOD, AND POST INTERVENTION TESTS (Standard
Deviations in parenthesis)

| | N = 7 TO 12 | | |
	PRE 1 INTERV.	PRE 2 INTERV.	POST INTERV.
Total Mood Score	27.3 (50.1)	18.4 (36.0)	0.0 (21.6)
Depression/ Dejection	12.8 (12.1)	10.9 (8.9)	6.4 (7.2)
Anger/ Hostility	9.5 (11.2)	9.7 (11.3)	7.4 (7.4)
Tension/ Anxiety	8.4 (7.8)	8.4 (6.9)	4.0 (5.3)
Vigour/ Activity	14.7 (7.9)	13.8 (7.5)	19.7[**] (7.1)
Fatigue/ Inertia	10.6 (7.5)	11.0 (9.5)	7.8 (7.6)
Confusion/ Bewilderment	3.4 (5.6)	2.8 (4.3)	-0.3[*] (2.5)

[*] p < 0.05, [**] p < 0.003 Contrast average (Pre 1 and Pre
2) vs Post.

The results for subjects completing the POMS at baseline (PRE 1), post intervention (POST) and six weeks after the intervention (FOLLOW UP) are presented in Table 4. There was a consistently significant difference between the average of the post intervention scores (POST and FOLLOW UP) compared to the pre intervention scores (PRE 1) for all the POMS dimensions and the TMS with p values ranging from < 0.05 to 0.0001. There were no significant differences between the POST and FOLLOW UP scores indicating that the reduction in psychological stress persisted for six weeks after the intervention was completed.

IMMUNOLOGICAL RESULTS

Delayed Hypersensitivity Skin Tests (DHST): Sixty two subjects completed baseline DHST. The mean number of positive responses to the DHST was 1.9 SD(1.4), range 0 - 6, and the mean total induration score 7.9mm SD(6.2), range 0 - 24.5 mm. In comparison to DHST normative data from a sample of 119 Australians of similar age (Hickie and Hickie 1990, personal communication), subjects in this study scored well below the

TABLE 4. REPEATED MEASURES DESIGN 2: MEAN PROFILE OF MOOD STATES (POMS) SCORES FOR PRE AND POST INTERVENTION AND 6 WEEK FOLLOW UP TESTS (Standard Deviations in parenthesis)

	PRE 1 INTERV.	N = 13 POST INTERV.	FOLLOW UP
Total Mood Score	48.3 ** (43.8)	1.9 (29.0)	4.0 (24.3)
Depression/ Dejection	15.5 * (12.4)	5.9 (6.9)	6.9 (6.6)
Anger/ Hostility	12.8 ** (9.6)	4.9 (4.7)	4.7 (3.9)
Tension/ Anxiety	12.4 * (8.4)	2.2 (6.2)	3.7 (6.2)
Vigour/ Activity	13.5 *** (6.5)	19.0 (7.6)	19.8 (7.6)
Fatigue/ Inertia	14.3 ** (9.2)	5.9 (6.4)	6.5 (4.5)
Confusion/ Bewilderment	6.7 ** (4.8)	2.0 (2.7)	2.0 (3.6)

* $p < 0.05$, ** $p < 0.02$, *** $p < 0.0001$, Contrast Pre 1 vs average (Post and Follow up).

'normal' level of 3.3 for the mean number of positive responses and 15.3mm for the mean total induration scorer. There was also a positive and significant correlation in our sample between age and the number of positive responses ($r = 0.34$, $p < 0.05$), which is consistent with results from previous studies.[20]

The 'within subjects design' results are presented in Table 5. Paired t-test comparisons of the 41 subjects completing pre and post intervention DHST scores revealed an almost statistically significant improvement in the number of positive responses after the intervention period ($p < 0.07$), while, for the control group, there was no significant difference. For the total induration score, results show there was no significant change over the six week period for either the control or intervention groups.

The Case-Control results shown in Table 6 illustrate that there was no significant difference between the amount each group changed over the 6 week period for either parameter of the DHST.

TABLE 5. GROUP MEANS FOR THE WITHIN SUBJECTS DESIGN: SUBJECTS COMPLETING PRE AND POST INTERVENTION AND CONTROL PERIOD DELAYED HYPERSENSITIVITY SKIN TESTS (standard deviations in parenthesis)

NUMBER OF POSITIVE RESPONSES (paired t-test)

	PRE	POST
CONTROL GROUP N=25	2.0 (1.6)	2.1 (1.5)
INTERVENTION GROUP N=41	1.9 (1.5)	2.3 (1.5)

TOTAL INDURATION SCORE (mm)

CONTROL GROUP N=25	8.2 (7.0)	8.7 (6.9)
INTERVENTION GROUP N=41	7.9 (6.6)	8.1 (6.3)

TABLE 6. GROUP MEANS FOR THE CASE-CONTROL DESIGN: INTERVENTION AND CONTROL GROUP DELAYED HYPERSENSITIVITY SKIN TESTS (standard deviations in parenthesis)

NUMBER OF POSITIVE RESPONSES (MANOVA)

	PRE	POST
CONTROL GROUP N = 25	2.0 (1.6)	2.1 (1.5)
INTERVENTION GROUP N = 24	1.8 (1.3)	2.2 (1.5)

TOTAL INDURATION SCORE (mm)

	PRE	POST
CONTROL GROUP N = 25	8.2 (7.0)	8.7 (6.9)
INTERVENTION GROUP N = 24	7.1 (5.6)	7.8 (6.1)

Results for the 17 subjects that 'crossed-over' from the six week control period into the intervention program are shown in Table 7. There were no statistically significant differences between the two control period and post intervention scores for either parameter of the DHST. However, there was a trend for an increase in the number of positive responses after the intervention period, ($p < 0.12$).

TABLE 7. REPEATED MEASURES DESIGN 1: MEAN PRE AND POST CONTROL PERIOD, AND POST INTERVENTION FOR THE DELAYED HYPERSENSITIVITY SKIN TESTS. (standard deviations in parenthesis).

N = 17	Number of Positive Reactions	Total Induration Score (mm)
Pre 1 Intervention	2.1 (1.8)	8.9 (7.9)
Pre 2 Intervention	2.0 (1.6)	8.7 (6.9)
Post intervention	2.5 (1.5)	8.7 (6.6)

TABLE 8. REPEATED MEASURES DESIGN 2: MEAN PRE AND POST INTERVENTION, AND FOLLOW UP RESULTS FOR THE DELAYED HYPERSENSITIVITY SKIN TESTS. (standard deviations in parenthesis)

	Number of Positive Reactions	Total Induration Score (mm)
Pre Intervention	1.4a (1.6)	4.9 (5.0)
Post Intervention	2.3 (1.4)	7.9b (6.3)
Follow Up	2.3 (1.4)	5.7 (4.9)

a $p < 0.05$ Contrasting Pre vs average (Post and Follow up).
b $p < 0.04$ post hoc comparison of Pre and Post scores.

Results for the 12 subjects completing the intervention and 6 week follow up tests are shown in Table 8. For the number of positive responses there was a statistically significant increase after the intervention, (p < 0.04), and this was maintained at 6 week follow up tests. For the total induration score there was a trend for increase after the intervention, (p < 0.13), contrasting pre with the average of post and follow up scores. There was also a trend for a return to base line levels at 6 week follow up tests, (p < 0.17, contrasting post with follow up). A *post hoc* analysis revealed that the post intervention total induration score significantly increased in comparison to the pre score (p < 0.04).

Phytohaemaglutinin (PHA) Mitogen Stimulation of Lymphocytes: Of the 63 subjects that were entered into the study pre and post intervention PHA tests were conducted on 29. The reduction in the number of subjects tested was due to a number of reasons: 24 did not return for blood tests and 10 subjects had low lymphocyte counts, and therefore, there were not enough cells to conduct the PHA assay. There is also a reduction in the number of subjects tested at the highest PHA concentration (1.5 μg/ml), which was due to the introduction of this concentration after the study had commenced.

Since the inter-assay variability is high in this test (35%), samples from the same

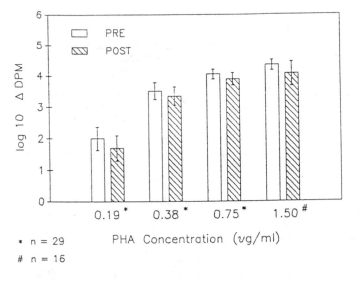

Figure 4. PHA stimulation of lymphocytes - Within subject design. Mean ($\pm$ SE) pre and post intervention scores for all subjects completing the intervention.

subjects were run together on the same plate at the same time. Hence, the statistical analyses conducted below, compares 'within subject' differences.

For the 'within subjects' design, paired t-test were conducted for each concentration of PHA. Results for the intervention group are presented in Figure 4. There was a statistically significant decrease in lymphocyte responsiveness for the 0.75 µg/ml PHA concentration in the intervention group (p < 0.04). However, for the other PHA concentrations there were no significant changes. For the control subjects, results presented in Figure 5 demonstrate that there was no significant differences between the two control period results. For the 'case-control design', change scores were calculated for the intervention and control subjects by subtracting pre scores from post scores, (Post - Pre). Positive values indicate improvement in lymphocyte responsiveness and vice versa. The mean change scores presented in Table 9, indicate that there were no consistent changes for either the control or intervention groups. Independent t-tests showed no statistical differences between the intervention and control groups for any of the four concentrations of PHA.

Results for subjects completing the pre and post 6 week control period and post intervention tests revealed that for the 0.75 µg/ml PHA concentration there was a significant decrease after the intervention compared to the mean of the wait list control values, (p < 0.04), while for the other PHA concentrations there were no significant differences. Results for subjects completing the intervention and then six week follow up tests showed a significant

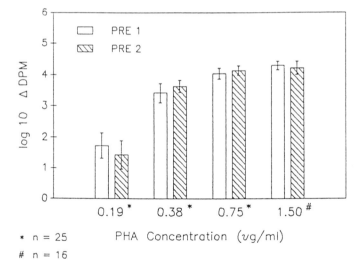

Figure 5. PHA stimulation of lymphocytes - Within subject design. Mean (± SE) control group scores pre (Pre 1) and post (Pre 2) the six week waiting period.

TABLE 9. CASE-CONTROL DESIGN: MEAN PHA MITOGEN STIMULATION CHANGE SCORES FOR THE INTERVENTION AND CONTROL GROUPS (standard deviations in parenthesis).

| | PHA concentration (ug/ml) | | | |
	0.19	0.38	0.75	1.50
Units: $\log_{10}$ DPM				
INTERVENTION GROUP N = 25,				
	-0.4	-0.1	-0.0	0.1^{n}
	(2.0)	(0.4)	(0.2)	(0.2)
CONTROL GROUP N = 18,				
	-0.3	0.2	0.1	$-0.1^{\#}$
	(2.0)	(1.2)	(0.4)	(0.5)

^{n} N = 16; $^{\#}$ N = 9.

decline in lymphocyte responsiveness after the intervention, (p < 0.05) which was maintained at follow up for the $0.19\mu g/ml$ PHA concentration. For the other PHA concentrations there were no significant differences between the average of post intervention and follow up scores compared to pre intervention scores, or between pre intervention compared to post intervention scores (Results not shown).

V. DISCUSSION

The 63 subjects entered into the study were a self selective group, and no conclusions can be drawn about how representative they were of the generality of friends and relatives of cancer patients. In addition, one third dropped out over the course of the study. Of those who completed tests, it can be seen from the high percentage of attendance and frequency of meditation practice, that these subjects were highly motivated, and committed to the intervention program. Hence the effects of such motivation must be taken into account, and caution must be exercised against generalisation of these results to the wider population of spouses of cancer patients. On the other hand, previous intervention studies have shown immuno-enhancement in a healthy geriatric sample,[6] and in medical students.[7] Therefore this type of intervention may be applicable to other psychologically distressed groups. In addition, this type of intervention may prove to be beneficial to cancer patients themselves.[21,22]

That the subjects were distressed was confirmed by their baseline GHQ scores which greatly exceeded those of a sample of 753 healthy Australians.[12] The GHQ is a well validated screening questionnaire for nonpsychotic psychiatric illness. Study subjects' baseline GHQ scores were significantly greater than published normative data, with the mean score being greater than the cut off level for "caseness", indicating that most subjects suffered unequivocal psychological distress.

On the basis of baseline delayed hypersensitivity skin test (DHST) scores, the subjects were also shown to be immune suppressed when compared to a sample of healthy Australian subjects of similar age (Hickie and Hickie, personal communication). The extensive use of medication in these subjects may have been a confounding factor, although the role of medication in altering immunity remains unclear. Pre and post assessments indicated that medication use did not change appreciably over the intervention and control periods. It should also be noted that if medication effects on immune function were suppressive, than it would only serve to weaken the effects of the intervention. Furthermore, the coexistence of low levels of immune function and psychological distress demonstrated in this study are consistent with findings of similar relationships in previous studies,[1] and more specifically, one previous study has shown that the care givers of the chronically ill are both psychologically and immunologically depressed.[9]

There were highly statistically significant improvements in the Profile Of Mood States (POMS) dimensions after the intervention period. The POMS scale consists of six dimensions and a total mood score (TMS) giving an overall profile of mood states. At baseline, subject's POMS scores were comparable to those of distressed psychiatric patients[14] but after the intervention fell to well below this level, indicating the effectiveness of the intervention program in reducing negative mood states, such as depression and anxiety. The improvement in psychological well-being after the group program could be explained in a number of ways, apart from attributing it to the specific effects of the intervention. The questionnaires used in this study have been shown to have adequate validity, reliability and internal consistency. However factors that may have affected subjects' scores include, inter alia, fatigue (there were 8 pages of questions), social desirability influences, expectancy effects and placebo effects.

The delayed hypersensitivity skin tests (DHST) measure in vivo cell mediated immunity, with increases in the number of positive responses and total induration scores indicating improved immune function. There were statistically significant changes in both measures of Delayed Hypersensitivity, with the total induration score and the number of positive responses both significantly increasing after the intervention for the group of subjects completing six week follow up tests. Also, for the number of positive responses, there was a trend towards an increased response in the other two univariate analyses, but the Case-Control analysis showed no significant difference. All other analyses for the total induration score showed no significant changes over the intervention period. An important variable that was not controlled for was the possible influence of intercurrent illness during the study. However, if the subjects did contract an illness during the study this would be expected to impair the immune response and therefore cause a decrease in the number of positive responses which would only serve to weaken the effects of the intervention. Other factors known to effect immune function such as sleep loss, weight loss, alcohol consumption, and cigarette smoking[11] did not significantly change over the course of the study, nor were there any self reported changes in medication use by subjects.

All the DHST scores were read by the same researcher, who was blind to the group allocation of subjects, except in a few cases where they informed the researcher of their status. The investigator was aware of the hypothesis of the research but it is unlikely that this affected the scoring as the two DHST measures did not covary, yet both were measured by the same research team member.

Since the results for changes in the number of positive responses and the total induration score are small and were not consistently found in all the analyses, they can only be regarded as suggestive of the possibility that the intervention programs may have improved *in vivo* immune function. The value of a repeat measures design using subjects as their own control should, however, be noted, since it is not as prey to the many sources of variance intrinsic to a case-control design, especially where there are small numbers of subjects. In this light, it is of interest that interpretable changes in CMI were most evident in the small number of subjects who completed the repeat measures tests. It is possible that where there were strong trends for an increase in the number of positive responses and little change in the total induration score that subjects may have become more sensitive to the different types of antigens as measured by the number of positive responses, but not in their overall reaction to the antigen, as measured by the total induration score. It is unlikely that the improved sensitivity to the antigens was due to inoculation as there were no significant changes seen in the control group, and also, this test has been demonstrated not to immunise subjects after repeated testing. The clinical significance of the changes in the number of positive responses and total induration score is unknown, and the mean increase was only in the order of 0.5 and 5 mm respectively. Future research will first need to replicate such changes before attempting to determine their clinical significance.

The PHA mitogen stimulation tests show a statistically significant decrease in *in vitro* lymphocyte function after the intervention for two concentrations of PHA, while no changes were detected over the 6 week control period. As previously noted, this type of immune test is susceptible to minor changes in experimental procedures. To reduce these effects, the cells were cyropreserved so that samples from each subject could be run at the same time. Although the cryopreservation procedure may alter the cells' function, and therefore make it difficult to draw inferences about *in vivo* immune function, this procedure was considered necessary on the basis of preliminary PHA assay results which showed a large inter-assay coefficient of variability.

Presuming the PHA results do reflect a decrease in lymphocyte function *in vivo*, they do conflict with those obtained from the in vivo immune tests. Both tests are thought to measure helper T-lymphocyte function, although assessing different aspects, and under different conditions. The PHA test measures T helper lymphocyte responsiveness to a "non specific" challenge in cell culture, and is considered a broad index of T lymphocyte function.[23] The DHST measures the *in vivo* memory capacity of T helper cells to recall antigens and, although it also provides a general overall measure of *in vivo* immune function,[20] a review of relevant studies reveals that there is no consistent association between *in vivo* and *in vitro* tests of lymphocyte function.[16,23]

Considering the results the study as a whole, although there were statistically significant changes in some immune parameters over the intervention, it cannot be concluded that the intervention exerted a general enhancing effect on lymphocyte function, and for this reason future studies will be necessary to resolve this question. It will be necessary to design studies with larger numbers of subjects, medication use will have to be controlled for, as will prevalence of intercurrent illness, and more extensive measures of immune function should be used.

Although the specific effects of each component of the intervention were not studied (meditation, relaxation and group discussion), the results are consistent with previous anecdotal evidence of Meares,[21] who noted reductions in anxiety in cancer patients following the practice of meditation. Furthermore, relaxation has been shown to improve psychological well-being,[6] and provision of social support (group discussion) to "buffer" against psychological stress.[1,24] However, there is a further need to determine which components of the intervention were most effective so that the practical and theoretical issues can be clarified. Such future studies may lead to a more effective and economical type of intervention. Also these results are tantalizing enough to warrant future research into the effects of psychological interventions on immune functions, and the clinical significance of such effects in changing the course of disease. One of the present limitations is lack of detailed knowledge about lymphocyte function and future work, for example, in the area of cytokines may provide more sensitive indicators of such functions.

Consideration should also be given to the clinical utility of providing such group interventions more widely for helping the relatives of cancer patients in general, as they have been shown in this (albeit in this instance in a self selected sample) and other studies to be psychologically distressed. Similarly the number of patients suffering psychological distress associated with having cancer, represents a substantial number of people, and this type of intervention may prove beneficial in helping them cope with the drastic changes occurring in their lives. Since it is a group program, it is cost-effective and could be seen as a practical adjuvant treatment for cancer patients and their families. More longitudinal studies need to be conducted in this area to further investigate the long-term psychological and physical outcomes of such treatment programmes for defined groups of chronically ill patients.

While acknowledging the possible confounding influences of expectancy and social desirability effects, it appears that the intervention program had a substantial impact on alleviating the psychological distress in these subjects. Whether this type of intervention can be used for other distressed populations is of considerable interest, since the group approach constitutes an efficient method for treating large numbers of patients. To achieve maximum improvement in psychological well-being in the most economic manner, future studies should be directed towards determining the effective components of such multimodal group interventions.

VI. ACKNOWLEDGEMENTS

Financial support for this study was provided by the NH&MRC and the St. George Hospital Cancer Research Fund.

VII. REFERENCES

1. Kiecolt-Glaser, J.K., Ricker, D., George, J., Nessick, G., Speicher, C.E., Garner, W. and Glaser, R., Urinary cortisol levels, cellual immunocompetence, and loneliness in psychiatric inpatients, *Psychosom.Med.*, 46, 15, 1984.

2. O'Donnell, M., Silove, D. and Wakefield, D., Current perspectives on immunology and psychiatry, *Aust.N.Z.J.Psychiatr.*, 22, 366, 1988.

3. Peavey, B.S., Lawlis, G.F. and Goven, A., Biofeedback-assisted relaxation: Effects on phagocytic capacity, *Biofeedback Self Regul.*, 10(1), 33, 1985.

4. Smith, G.R. and McDaniel, S.M., Psychologically mediated effect on the delayed hypersensitivity reaction to Tuberculin in humans, *Psychosom.Med.*, 45, 65, 1983.

5. Rider, M.S. and Achterberg, J., Effect of music-assisted imagery on neutrophils and lymphocytes, *Biofeedback Self Regul.*, 14(3), 247, 1989.

6. Kiecolt-Glaser, J.K., Glaser, R., Willinger, D., Stout, J., Messick, G., Sheppard, S., Ricker, D., Romisher, S.C., Briner, W., Bonnell, G. and Donnerberg, R., Psychosocial enhancement of immunocompetence in a geriatric population, *Health Psychology*, 4(1), 25, 1985.

7. Kiecolt-Glaser, J.K., Glaser, R., Strain, E.C., Stout, J.C., Tarr, K.L., Holliday, J.E. and Speicher, C.E., Modulation of cellular immunity in medical students, *J.Behav.Med.*, 9, 5, 1986.

8. Lewis, F.M., Strengthening family supports. Cancer and the family, *Cancer*, 65, 752, 1990.

9. Kiecolt-Glaser, J.K., Glaser, R., Shuttleworth, E.C., Dyer, C.S., Ogrocki, P. and Speicher, C.E., Chronic stress and immunity in family caregivers of Alzheimer's disease victims, *Psychosom.Med.*, 49, 523, 1987.

10. Rabins, P.V., Fitting, N.D., Eastham, J. and Fetting, J., The emotional impact of caring for the chronically ill, *Psychosomatics*, 31(3), 331, 1990.

11. Kiecolt-Glaser, J.K. and Glaser, R., Methodological issues in behavioural immunology research with humans, *Brain Behav.Immun.*, 2, 67, 1988.

12. Goodchild, M.E. and Duncan-Jones, P., Chronicity and the General Health Questionnire, *Br.J.Psychiatr.*, 146, 55, 1985.

13. Tarnopolosky, A., Hand, D.J., NcLean, E.R., Roberts, H. and Wiggins, R.D., Validity and uses of a screening questionnaire (GHQ) in the community, *Br.J.Psychiatr.*, 134, 508, 1979.

14. McNair, D.M., Lorr, N.L. and Droppleman, L.F., *Edits Manual for the Profile of Mood States*, Edits, San Diego, California, 1981.

15. Linn, B.S. and Jensen, J., Age and immune suppression to a surgical stress, *Archs.Surgery*, 118, 405, 1983.

16. Bartrop, R.W., Luckhurst, E., Lazarus, L.D., Kiloh, L.G. and Penny, R., Depressed lymphocyte function after bereavement, *Lancet*, 1, 834, 1977.

17. Schleifer, S.J., Reller, S.E., Meyerson, A.T., Raskin, N.J., Davis, R.L. and Stein, M., Lymphocyte function in major depressive disorder, *Archs Gen.Psychiatry*, 41, 484, 1984.

18. Maluish, A. and Strong, D., Lymphocyte proliferation, in *Manual of clinical laboratory immunology*, Rose, N., Friedman, H. and Fahey, J., Eds., American Society for Microbiology, Washington, 1986. 274.

19. Golub, S.H., Cryopreservation of Human Lymphocytes, in *In Vitro Methods in Cell-Mediated and Tumor Immunity*, Bloom, B.R. and David, J.R., Eds., 1985.

20. Kniker, W.T., Anderson, C.T. and Roumiantzeff, M., The multi-test system: A standardized approach to evaluation of delayed hypersensitivity and cell mediated immunity, *Ann.Allergy*, 43, 73, 1979.

21. Meares, A., Regression of recurrence of carcinoma of the breast at mastectomy site associated with intensive meditation, *Aust.Fam.Phys.*, 10, 218, 1981.

22. Spiegel, D., Bloom, J., Braemer, H. and Gottheil, E., Effect of psychosocial treatment on survival of patients with metastatic breast cancer, *Lancet*, ii, 888, 1989.

23. Graybill, J.R. and Alford, R.H., Variability of sequential studies of lymphocyte blastogenesis in normal adults, *Clin.Exp.Immunol.*, 25, 28, 1976.

24. Thomas, P.D., Goodwin, J.N. and Goodwin, J.S., Effect of social support on stress-related changes in cholesterol level, uric acid level, and immune function in an elderly sample, *Am.J.Psychiatr.*, 735, 1985.

IMMUNE DYSFUNCTION IN DEPRESSIVE DISORDERS

Ian Hickie[a], and Catherine Hickie[b]

[a]Mood Disorders Unit, Prince Henry Hospital, Sydney,
and [b] New South Wales Institute of Psychiatry

In the field of immune dysfunction in depressive disorders there are three important considerations. Firstly, are there detectable immune abnormalities in patients with depressive disorders? Secondly, if such abnormalities are present, are they medically significant? Finally, if immune abnormalities are present in patients when they are depressed, are they reversible following effective treatment of the depressive episode? We will deal with each of these questions and present aspects of our own research which have targeted specifically the first and third questions.

There is already a public belief that strong scientific evidence exists to support the proposition that depressed mood is associated with immune impairment. In a survey of our final year medical students (n = 116, median age 23 years) during 1990, 95% of respondents believed that depression increased a person's chance of becoming medically ill while 71% asserted that immunodeficiency was a likely mechanism of this increased morbidity. Eighty-seven per cent reported that depression resulted in medically significant immune dysfunction, although only 21% were able to offer a plausible pathophysiology as to how this might occur.

Although a number of research reports over the last decade have suggested an association between depressive disorders and impaired cell-mediated immunity (CMI), especially in older more severely depressed patients, the results have been inconsistent.[1] It would seem premature, to us, to conclude that the association had been clearly demonstrated. The apparent inconsistencies, in particular with regard to immune abnormalities in less severely depressed outpatients, may reflect limitations in the breadth of assessment of immune functions and a failure to examine for the possible differential effects of subtypes of depression. Notably, in the largest study yet published, Schleifer et al[2] found no differences in CMI measures between 91 patients with major depression and normal control subjects, matched for age and sex. The patients in that study were mainly young female outpatients and the potential relevance of sub-types of depression was not examined.

Our review of the available literature[1] suggested that disturbance of CMI may be limited largely to with melancholic rather than non-melancholic disorders. Theoretically, a number of other features which are characteristic of melancholia (such as significant weight loss, hypercortisolaemia, increased catecholamine turnover and disturbed sleep architecture) may explain such a link to impaired CMI. To demonstrate that disturbance of CMI is directly related to the diagnosis of melancholia, it is essential to compare such patients not only with other depressive subtypes, but also with sex and age-matched normal control subjects.

Previous research has focused on *in vitro* techniques. It seems more clinically relevant to broaden assessment techniques to include *in vivo* measures. To that end, in our studies, we have focused on not only on the relevance of subtypes of depression, but also on the assessment of delayed-type hypersensidvity (DTH) skin responses to a panel of standard antigens. We have utilised a commercially-available DTH kit whose properties have been explored extensively in normal and medically-ill subjects.

In our initial case-control study we assessed CMI in 57 patients with major depression (31 with melancholic, 26 with non-melancholic disorders) and age and sex-matched controls by both *in vitro* and *in vivo* immunological techniques. Compared to control subjects and patients with non-melancholic depression patients with melancholia demonstrated reduced delayed-type hypersensitivity (DTH) skin responses and showed trends toward impaired lymphocyte proliferative responses to the mitogen phytohaemagglutinin (PHA). These data were supportive of our hypothesis that impairment of CMI in patients with depressive disorders may be limited to those with melancholia. Consequently, in answer to our first question of whether immune dysfunction is present in depressive disorders, our review and our own research would suggest that the proposition is only supported in a small subgroup of depressives who tend to be older, hospitalised, more severely depressed and tend to have a melancholic rather than non-melancholic depressive disorder.

Our second consideration is whether any recorded immune impairment in depressed patients is medically significant. Although we have not conducted any studies in this area ourselves, we will establish shortly a longitudinal examination of the proposition that immune impairment in patients with melancholia results in increased physical morbidity. Previous epidemiological studies suggest that patients with depressive disorders who have been

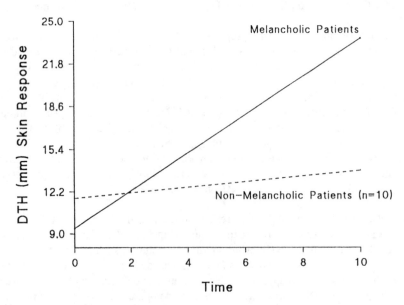

Figure 1. Change in DTH skin response after treatment. Melancholic patients (n=7) show significant improvement (p=0.03).

hospitalised or were older at the onset of their disorder have an increased standardised mortality ratio. No clear link, however, has been established with disorders that may be influenced by impaired immune competence such as infectious diseases or malignancies. In long-term prospective studies the presence of depressive *symptoms* rather than clinical depressive disorders, has not been clearly linked with an increased risk of malignancy. All studies of natural health outcomes in clinical populations of depressed patients are difficult as a result of the markedly increased death rate due to suicide. Only longitudinal studies assessing depression, immune function and physical health over a prolonged period are likely to answer the question of whether immune dysfunction in patients with depressive syndromes result in impaired physical health.

The third question, which we have started to address, is whether immune dysfunction in patients with depressive disorders is reversed by effective therapy. In a current longitudinal study 17 patients with depressive disorders who were unmedicated (except for benzodiazepines) at the baseline assessment were reviewed psychiatrically and immunologically after ten weeks. Effective psychiatric treatment resulted in normalization of the immune response, particularly in melancholic patients who have received pharmacotherapy (Figure 1).

This is particularly encouraging, as previous reports have suggested that antidepressants may have immunosuppressive properties. Non-melancholic patients were not impaired at baseline and, on the whole, did not receive pharmacotherapy. They have also experienced less change in their depressive symptoms over the course of the study. It would appear that effective pharmacotherapy for melancholic depressive disorders results in normalization of CMI as assessed by both DTH skin testing and PHA mitogen stimulation assay. Further research will seek to clarify the relationships between depressive sub-types, treatment, and immune outcomes over time.

I. REFERENCES

1.   Hickie, I., Silove, D., Hickie, C., Wakefield, D. and Lloyd, A., Is there immune dysfunction in depressive disorders ? *Psychol.Med.*, 20, 755, 1990.
2.   Schleifer, S.J., Keller, S.E., Bond, R.N., Cohen, J. and Stein, M., Major depressive disorder and immunity, *Arch.Gen.Psychiatry*, 46, 81, 1989.

Index

INDEX